MW01490448

THE SASS-BACK KITCHEN

SUE. B. SLAUGHTER

The Sass-Back Kitchen

Eat Bold, Feel Bright, Bloat No More and Tell Brain Fog to Buzz off

Sue B. Slaughter

© 2025 by Sue Slaughter.

All rights reserved. No part of this publication may be reproduced, distributed, or transmitted in any form or by any means, including photocopying, recording, or other electronic or mechanical methods, without the prior written permission of the publisher, except in the case of brief quotations embodied in critical reviews and certain other noncommercial uses permitted by copyright law.

CONTENTS

PREFACE

When you're told "your labs are normal," but you feel anything but...

When your joints ache, your skin flares, your belly bloats, and your energy disappears—but no one can tell you why...

When your daily reality is shaped by mysterious inflammation, autoimmune flares, chronic fatigue, or digestive distress—it's easy to feel hopeless.

You're not alone.

In fact, over 50 million Americans are living with autoimmune disease—and that number is rising every year. Millions more suffer from chronic inflammatory conditions like arthritis, eczema, fibromyalgia, migraines, and irritable bowel syndrome. And for many, food is both the trigger—and the answer.

More than 70% of our immune system lives in the gut. What we eat isn't just fuel—it's information. For those of us with hypersensitive systems, foods like gluten, dairy, soy, sugar, and highly processed oils can act like a match to dry grass, igniting everything from brain fog to full-body pain.

I know this not just as an author, but as a patient. For years, I lived in survival mode—cycling through specialists, elimination diets, and endless supplements—until I realized the most powerful medicine was in my own kitchen.

This book is born from that breakthrough.

The Sass-Back Kitchen is more than a cookbook—it's a permission slip to take control. It's a toolkit for anyone who's tired of flares dictating their life. It's for the woman who gave up bread and cried in the grocery aisle, unsure what to eat. For the man who's done with Band-Aid treatments and ready for root cause solutions. For the parents trying to feed their kids healing food without creating fear around it.

Inside, you'll find:

- Recipes free of gluten, dairy, soy, refined sugar, and artificial additives
- Nutrient-rich meals that support gut health, hormone balance, and immune regulation
- Comforting, colorful dishes that prove healing food can also be delicious
- A system to help you track how food makes you feel—and create your personalized healing blueprint

Most importantly, you'll find hope.

Healing is not a straight line. But every small change, every nourishing meal, every flare-free day adds up.

Let this book be your guide—and your cheerleader—as you reclaim your plate, your body, and your peace.

Because you deserve more than symptom management. You deserve to thrive.

PART ONE

The Anti-Inflammatory Plan That Works

1: Foods and Oils Safe for You

Food is one of the most powerful tools for fighting inflammation. The right foods and oils can soothe the body, reduce chronic inflammation, and improve overall health. But with so many options available, how do you know which are truly anti-inflammatory and beneficial to your health?

Let's start with the basics: which foods are anti-inflammatory? While there is no one-size-fits-all solution, certain foods are consistently shown to reduce inflammation. These foods are high in nutrients, antioxidants, and healthy fats, which help your body's natural healing processes. Here's a list of some of the best foods to incorporate into your anti-inflammatory diet:

1. Fruits
Fruits are high in vitamins, minerals, fiber, and antioxidants, which help fight inflammation. Some fruits outperform others in terms of anti-inflammatory properties:

- Berries (blueberries, strawberries, raspberries, and blackberries) are high in antioxidants called anthocyanins, which have been shown to reduce inflammation and protect cells from damage.
- Cherries: Tart cherries, which contain anthocyanins, have been linked to reduced inflammation, particularly in joint tissues.
- Apples: Apples, a high-fiber, antioxidant-rich food, help to reduce inflammation and promote gut health.
- Oranges: Oranges are high in vitamin C and flavonoids, which have natural anti-inflammatory properties and boost the immune system.
- Pineapple contains bromelain, an enzyme that reduces inflammation, particularly in the digestive system.

2] Vegetables

Vegetables are an essential component of the anti-inflammatory diet. Many are high in fiber, vitamins, and minerals, which help to reduce inflammation:

- Leafy Greens** (spinach, kale, Swiss chard, collard greens): High in antioxidants like vitamin K, these greens help reduce oxidative stress in the body.
- Broccoli: A cruciferous vegetable rich in sulforaphane, a potent anti-inflammatory compound.
- Bell Peppers: Bell peppers are high in vitamin C and have been shown to reduce inflammation, especially in the joints.
- Cauliflower: Another cruciferous vegetable that lowers inflammation and promotes overall health.
- Sweet Potatoes: A high-quality source of beta-carotene, an anti-inflammatory vitamin A.

3. Lean proteins

Not all proteins are created equal, and selecting the appropriate ones is critical for reducing inflammation. Lean proteins, which are low in unhealthy fats, help the body without causing inflammation:

- Fish: Fatty fish such as salmon, mackerel, sardines, and tuna are high in omega-3 fatty acids, which are known to reduce inflammation.
- Chicken and Turkey: Choose lean cuts, such as skinless breast meat, which provide high-quality protein without excessive saturated fat.
- Tofu and Tempeh: These plant-based proteins are anti-inflammatory, promote heart health, and reduce oxidative stress.
- Eggs: Eggs, particularly those from pasture-raised chickens, contain anti-inflammatory omega-3s.

4. Nuts and Seeds

Nuts and seeds are high in healthy fats, fiber, and antioxidants, making them an ideal snack on an anti-inflammatory diet. Some of the best are:

- Almonds: Rich in vitamin E, which reduces oxidative stress and inflammation.
- Walnuts: High in omega-3 fatty acids, which lower the body's inflammation markers.
- CHIA SEEDS: Chia seeds are an excellent plant-based source of omega-3s and fiber, making them ideal for smoothies or salads.
- Flax Seeds: Flaxseeds are high in lignans, which help with hormonal balance and inflammation.

5) Whole Grains

Whole grains, unlike refined grains, are high in fiber and antioxidants, which can help reduce inflammation. They help to regulate blood sugar, improve digestion, and promote heart health. The best whole grains for your anti-inflammatory diet are:

- Oats: A good source of beta-glucan fiber, which helps to reduce inflammation in the digestive system.
- Brown Rice: Packed with antioxidants and fiber, brown rice promotes healthy digestion and provides long-lasting energy.
- Quinoa: A protein-rich whole grain that also contains magnesium, which has anti-inflammatory properties.
- Barley: Barley contains antioxidants and fiber, which reduce inflammatory markers in the body.

Best Oils to Reduce Inflammation

Now that we've covered the foods you should eat, let's discuss oils. Oils are an important part of the anti-inflammatory diet because they contain essential fatty acids, which promote cellular health and reduce inflammation. These are the best oils to use:

1. Olive oil

In terms of anti-inflammatory properties, olive oil reigns supreme. It's high in monounsaturated fats, which have been linked to lower inflammation markers. Olive oil also contains polyphenols, which are antioxidants that protect the body's cells from oxidative stress.

- How to Use: Use extra virgin olive oil in salad dressings, drizzle over roasted vegetables, or add to cooked dishes at the end to enhance the flavor.

2. Avocado oil

Avocado oil is a healthy fat that contains monounsaturated fats and antioxidants. It also has a high smoke point, making it ideal for cooking at high temperatures.

- How to Use: Use avocado oil for stir-frying, grilling, or making homemade mayonnaise or salad dressings.

3) Coconut Oil

Coconut oil contains a high concentration of medium-chain triglycerides (MCTs), which can reduce inflammation and improve brain and heart health. While it's best used in moderation, it's an excellent choice for some recipes.

- How to Use: Coconut oil is ideal for baking, sautéing, and blending into smoothies for a creamy texture.

4) Flaxseed Oil

Flaxseed oil is high in omega-3 fatty acids, which are known to reduce inflammation. It also promotes heart health and hormonal balance.

- How to Use: Flaxseed oil works best in cold dishes, such as salad dressings, or drizzled over steamed vegetables. Avoid using it for high-heat cooking, as it may lose nutritional value.

5) Walnut Oil
Walnut oil, which contains omega-3 fatty acids and antioxidants, can help reduce inflammation and improve brain function.

- How to Use: Add walnut oil to salad dressings, drizzle it over roasted vegetables, or use it to finish pasta dishes.

Nutritional Advantages of These Foods and Oils

Incorporating these anti-inflammatory foods and oils into your diet provides your body with a variety of nutrients that can help reduce inflammation and promote healing. Here are some key advantages:

- Antioxidant-Rich: Many of these foods are high in antioxidants, which help protect the body's cells from free radical damage.
- Heart-Healthy Fats: Healthy fats found in foods such as olive oil, avocado, and nuts help lower LDL (bad) cholesterol and reduce the risk of cardiovascular disease.
- Reduced Joint Pain: Omega-3 fatty acids, found in fatty fish, walnuts, and flaxseed oil, have been shown to reduce joint inflammation and relieve arthritis symptoms.
- Improved Digestion: Fibre-rich foods, such as fruits, vegetables, and whole grains, promote healthy digestion and reduce gut inflammation.
- Brain Health: Many of these foods and oils, especially those high in omega-3s, can help protect the brain from inflammation and improve cognitive function.

How to Add These to Your Daily Meals

Incorporating anti-inflammatory foods and oils into your diet does not have to be difficult. Here are some simple ways to incorporate them into your daily routine:

- Begin your day with a smoothie: Combine berries, spinach, chia seeds, and a tablespoon of flaxseed or avocado oil for a delicious anti-inflammatory breakfast.
- Make salads your friend: Combine leafy greens, bell peppers, and avocado, then drizzle with olive oil and sprinkle with walnuts or flaxseeds.
- Cook with heart-healthy oils: When sautéing vegetables or grilling chicken, use olive or avocado oil. These oils enhance the flavor of your meals while also providing anti-inflammatory benefits.
- Snack on nuts: A handful of almonds or walnuts is a quick and simple anti-inflammatory snack.

- Include fish in your weekly menu: Aim for two to three servings of fatty fish each week. You can grill salmon, toss it in a salad, or make a simple fish taco with avocado and cilantro.

2: Foods and Oils Not For You

When you're trying to reduce inflammation and improve your health, one of the most important steps is to avoid foods and oils that can cause or worsen inflammation. While there is no doubt that incorporating the right foods into your diet can make a significant difference, eliminating the wrong ones is equally important.

Inflammatory Foods to Avoid

It's easy to become overwhelmed by all the "good" foods that combat inflammation, but what about the foods that cause it? A few foods and oils can cause inflammation, cell damage, and predispose you to future health issues. Let's break down the main culprits.

1. Processed food

Processed foods are those that have been altered in some way from their natural state, typically to increase shelf life or flavor. While convenient, they are often loaded with unhealthy fats, sugars, and additives that can cause inflammation.

- Avoid packaged snacks (chips, cookies, and crackers), frozen meals, and ready-to-eat processed meats such as hot dogs and deli meats.

These foods are frequently high in unhealthy fats, refined sugars, and sodium, which raises levels of inflammatory markers in the body. Over time, a processed food diet can cause chronic inflammation, weight gain, and an increased risk of heart disease, diabetes, and other health problems.

2. Refined sugars

Sugar may taste sweet, but it's not good for your body. Refined sugars are a major cause of inflammation.

- What to Avoid: Soda, candy, sugary desserts, breakfast cereals with added sugar, sugary fruit juices, and sweetened coffee drinks.

Refined sugars are quickly absorbed into the bloodstream, resulting in a blood sugar spike and the release of inflammatory substances. High sugar consumption also contributes to insulin resistance, which can cause additional inflammation and increase your risk of developing conditions such as type 2 diabetes and heart disease.

3. Transfats

Trans fats are artificial fats produced through a process known as hydrogenation, which solidifies liquid oils at room temperature. These fats were once common in many processed foods, but they are now prohibited in many places due to their negative effects.

- Avoid: Margarine, packaged baked goods (cookies, cakes, pastries), fried foods, and anything containing partially hydrogenated oils.

Trans fats are known to increase LDL (bad) cholesterol while decreasing HDL (good) cholesterol. This imbalance can cause inflammation in the arteries, raising the risk of heart disease, stroke, and other cardiovascular issues.

4) Refined Carbohydrates

Refined carbohydrates, such as white bread, pasta, and pastries, are derived from highly processed grains that have lost their nutrients and fiber.

- Avoid: White bread, pasta, white rice, baked goods containing white flour, and most breakfast cereals.

These foods digest quickly, resulting in spikes in blood sugar and insulin levels, which can cause inflammation. Over time, a refined carbohydrate diet can lead to weight gain, insulin resistance, and inflammation-related diseases such as arthritis and type 2 diabetes.

5. Omega-6-rich oils

While omega-6 fatty acids are necessary for good health, most people consume them in excess, which can cause inflammation. The key is to balance omega-6 intake with omega-3 fatty acids, but the typical Western diet is heavily reliant on omega-6-rich oils.

- Avoid: Vegetable oils such as soybean, corn, sunflower, and cottonseed oil. These are typically found in processed and fried foods.

Consuming too many omega-6 fatty acids and insufficient omega-3 fatty acids can disrupt your body's balance, resulting in chronic inflammation. Inflammation is linked to a wide range of chronic diseases, including heart disease, cancer, and autoimmune disorders.

6. Artificial additives and preservatives

Many processed foods contain artificial additives and preservatives that improve flavor, color, and shelf life. While these may appear to be harmless, they can have a negative long-term impact on your health.

- Avoid: Artificial sweeteners (such as aspartame and sucralose), MSG (monosodium glutamate), and food colorings.

According to some studies, artificial additives can cause inflammatory responses in the body, potentially leading to food sensitivities or worsening conditions such as asthma, migraines, and irritable bowel syndrome (IBS).

7. Alcohol (excess)
While a glass of wine or a beer on occasion may not be harmful, excessive alcohol consumption has been shown to increase inflammation.

- What to Avoid: Too much alcohol (more than one drink per day for women, two drinks per day for men).

Alcohol can irritate the gut, upset the balance of gut bacteria, and raise inflammatory markers. Over time, heavy drinking can cause liver damage, cardiovascular disease, and gastrointestinal issues.

The Bad Effects of These Foods on Your Health

Consuming these inflammatory foods can have a range of detrimental effects on your body, including:

- Chronic Inflammation: These foods can promote long-term, low-grade inflammation, which has been linked to a number of health issues, including arthritis, heart disease, diabetes, and even certain types of cancer.
- Weight Gain: Many of these foods contain a lot of calories but very little nutrition. Eating too many processed or sugary foods can cause weight gain, which contributes significantly to inflammation
- Gut Health Issues: Consuming refined sugars, unhealthy fats, and artificial additives can disrupt the delicate balance of bacteria in your gut, resulting in digestive problems and a weakened immune system.
- Heart Disease: Trans fats, refined sugars, and omega-6 oils all contribute to heart disease by raising bad cholesterol, increasing blood pressure, and causing arterial inflammation.
- Insulin Resistance: Excess sugar and refined carbohydrate consumption can cause insulin resistance, a condition in which the body's cells do not respond properly to insulin. This can eventually result in type 2 diabetes and other metabolic disorders.

Strategies to Eliminate or Replace These Foods

Now that we've covered which foods to avoid and why, let's look at some practical strategies for eliminating or replacing these inflammatory foods in your diet. With a little planning and creativity, you can make healthier choices that don't leave you feeling deprived.

1. Swap Processed Snacks for Whole Foods
Instead of eating packaged chips, cookies, or crackers, opt for whole, nutrient-dense snacks such as fresh fruit, nuts, seeds, or homemade energy bars. Prepare healthy snacks ahead of time so you always have something to grab when you get hungry.

2. Replace refined sugar with natural sweeteners
Are you craving something sweet? Instead of refined sugar, use natural sweeteners such as honey, maple syrup, or stevia. You can also satisfy your sweet tooth by eating fresh fruit or a small piece of dark chocolate (at least 70% cocoa). Remember that even with natural sweeteners, moderation is key.

3. Select Healthy Fats over Trans Fats
When cooking, use healthy oils such as olive, avocado, or coconut oil. If you want something creamy, swap out butter for avocado or hummus. When shopping, check the labels for trans fats in packaged foods and select products that are free of partially hydrogenated oils.

4. Replace refined carbs with whole grains
Instead of white bread or pasta, choose whole grains such as quinoa, brown rice, whole wheat bread, and whole grain pasta. Whole grains are packed with fiber, which helps regulate blood sugar and supports overall gut health. If you're new to whole grains, start with one or two, such as oats or brown rice, and gradually add more.

5. Reduce your alcohol consumption
Moderation is key when it comes to alcohol consumption. Limit your alcohol intake to one or two drinks per day, and stay hydrated with water throughout the day. If you find it difficult to cut back, try having alcohol-free days or switching to lighter drinks like spritzers or wine with sparkling water.

6. Learn how to read labels
Many processed foods contain hidden sugars, unhealthy fats, and artificial ingredients. Learn to read food labels so you can avoid products with unnecessary ingredients. Look for items that have been minimally processed and contain whole food ingredients.

7. Meal Prep and Planning
Planning your meals ahead of time can help you avoid the temptation to consume unhealthy processed foods. Spend some time each week preparing meals, snacks, and ingredients to ensure you always have healthy options available.

3: Best Cooking Methods

Sue Slaughter

When it comes to eating an anti-inflammatory diet, how you prepare your food is equally important as what you eat. The cooking methods you use can either preserve or destroy the nutrients in your food. To get the most out of your anti-inflammatory meals, use techniques that retain nutrients while also promoting the health benefits of the ingredients you're using.

There are several cooking methods that are especially beneficial for keeping your food nutritious, flavorful, and anti-inflammatory. The goal is to avoid methods that use a lot of added fats or oils while still preserving the vitamins, minerals, and antioxidants in your food.

1. Steaming

Steaming is one of the healthiest cooking methods because it uses water vapor to cook food, preserving the majority of its nutrients. Steamed vegetables, in particular, retain more of their water-soluble vitamins, such as vitamin C and vitamin B, which are otherwise lost during high-heat cooking methods.

- Benefits: Steaming preserves nutrients, uses little to no added fat, and can be done quickly. It works especially well with delicate foods such as vegetables, fish, and some grains.
- Best for: Vegetables (such as broccoli, spinach, and carrots), fish, and even fruits (for a warm, soft dessert, try pears or apples).

2. Grilling

Grilling is another excellent cooking method that imparts flavor to food without requiring excessive oils or fats. It is a dry-heat method in which food is cooked over an open flame, usually on a grill. Grilling can be a tricky method for preserving food's anti-inflammatory properties, but when done correctly, it can be very healthy.

- Benefits: Grilling allows excess fat to drain from food, making it an excellent choice for lean meats. It also helps to lock in flavors, and the charred effect (from grilling) can give your food a rich, smoky flavor without adding sugar or unhealthy fats.
- Perfect for: Lean meats (chicken, turkey, fish), vegetables (such as zucchini, peppers, and asparagus), and even fruits (like pineapple or peaches).

3) Baking

Baking is another great cooking method that allows you to prepare food without using unhealthy fats. It is done with dry heat in an oven and works well for everything from vegetables to proteins to baked goods (just make sure they are made with healthy ingredients!).

- Benefits: Baking retains moisture in food and requires little added fat. It is ideal for cooking large quantities of food at once, as well as batch cooking.

- Perfect for vegetables (sweet potatoes, cauliflower, squash), lean meats (chicken, turkey breast), and whole grains (quinoa, brown rice). Fish can also be baked, particularly if it is wrapped in parchment paper and seasoned with herbs and spices.

4) Sautéing

Sautéing is a quick cooking technique that involves cooking food in a small amount of fat (such as olive oil or avocado oil) over medium-high heat. This method is best suited for foods that cook quickly and do not require extended cooking times.

- Benefits: Sautéing requires little fat and is ideal for preserving the flavor of your ingredients. Sautéing with heart-healthy oils like olive or avocado oil can be a very healthy way to cook.
- Best for: Vegetables (spinach, mushrooms, or bell peppers), lean proteins (chicken, fish, tofu), and whole grains (quinoa or farro).

5) Roasting

Roasting is the process of cooking food in an oven over dry heat at high temperatures (usually 400°F or higher). It is similar to baking, but often done at a higher temperature to achieve a crispy exterior.

- Benefits: Roasting helps caramelize the natural sugars in vegetables, bringing out rich flavors without adding any additional sugar or fat. It's a simple method that results in a lot of flavor.
- Best for: Vegetables (sweet potatoes, Brussels sprouts, carrots, beets), chicken, and seafood.

6. Poaching

Poaching is a gentle cooking method that involves simmering food in a liquid such as water, broth, or even wine. It's ideal for delicate foods like eggs and fish because it retains their flavors and moisture.

- Benefits: Poaching is a low-fat cooking method that uses liquid to infuse food with flavor. It also preserves moisture, which aids in nutrient retention.
- Perfect for: Fish, eggs, fruit (like pears or apples), and lean meats like chicken.

7. Slow Cooking

Slow cooking, whether done in a slow cooker or an instant pot, is a method of cooking food for an extended period of time on low heat. It is ideal for preparing stews, soups, and other one-pot meals.

- Benefits: Slow cooking allows flavors to develop gradually and tenderizes tougher cuts of meat without using excessive fats or oils. It's ideal for meal prepping and cooking large quantities of food.
- Perfect for soups, stews, chili, and lean meats (such as chicken breast or lean beef).

Cooking Techniques to Preserve Food's Anti-Inflammatory Properties

Not all cooking methods are created equal when it comes to preserving your food's anti-inflammatory properties. To ensure you get the most out of your ingredients, here are a few tips for maximizing their health benefits while cooking:

1. Apply low to medium heat
When cooking, especially with vegetables and lean proteins, avoid using extremely high temperatures. Overheating food can destroy sensitive nutrients, such as vitamin C in vegetables, and produce toxic compounds, such as acrylamide in starchy foods. To preserve your food's anti-inflammatory properties, cook at low to medium heat whenever possible.

2. Keep It Simple with Healthy Fats
While healthy fats such as olive oil, avocado oil, and coconut oil can improve the flavor and nutrient absorption of your meals, they should not be used excessively. Use fats sparingly and select those that can withstand moderate heat, such as extra virgin olive oil, when sautéing or roasting. Remember: a little goes a long way!

3. Steam, Do Not Boil
Steaming is an excellent method for cooking vegetables because it preserves their water-soluble vitamins. When you boil vegetables, their nutrients leach into the water and are frequently discarded. Steaming, on the other hand, allows the vegetables to keep the majority of their nutritional value.

4. Use Herbs and Spices
Incorporating anti-inflammatory spices such as turmeric, ginger, garlic, and cinnamon into your cooking not only adds flavor but also improves the nutritional value of your meals. These spices are high in antioxidants and can help reduce inflammation. Sprinkle them on your meals or cook with them to infuse them with anti-inflammatory properties.

5. Avoid overcooking
Overcooking food, particularly vegetables, can reduce nutritional value and cause the breakdown of beneficial compounds. To maintain their anti-inflammatory properties, cook vegetables just until tender but still vibrant and crisp. Aim for al dente vegetables over mushy ones.

Tips for Meal Planning and Cooking for Busy Lifestyles

When you're busy, it's tempting to eat processed, unhealthy foods or order takeout. However, with a little planning, you can quickly and easily prepare anti-inflammatory meals. Here are some tips for meal prepping and cooking while on the go:

1. Plan Your Meals Ahead

Meal planning is essential for eating healthily on a busy schedule. Spend some time each week (usually on the weekend) planning your meals for the following days. This will help you avoid making last-minute unhealthy choices and ensure that you have everything you need to prepare nutritious meals. Try to keep your meals simple, using only a few key ingredients for various recipes.

2. Batch-cook and freeze
If you have a busy week ahead, try batch cooking and freezing your meals. Soups, stews, and casseroles can be made in large batches and portioned out for easy meals throughout the week. Just reheat and enjoy!

3. Prepare ingredients
Rather than preparing entire meals ahead of time, try prepping ingredients ahead. Wash and chop vegetables, marinate proteins, and prepare grains like quinoa or rice in bulk. When you're ready to cook, you'll be able to put everything together quickly.

4. Using a Slow Cooker or Instant Pot
These appliances are a lifesaver on busy days. You can put all of your ingredients in, set it, and forget it. Dinner will be ready when you arrive home. Slow cookers and instant pots are ideal for preparing soups, stews, and even large batches of beans or grains.

5. Keep Healthy Snacks on Hand
Stock your kitchen with healthy, convenient snacks such as nuts, fruit, yogurt, or hummus with vegetables. These snacks are ideal for busy days when you need something quick and nutritious to get you through.

4: Electrolyte Intake Routine

When it comes to an anti-inflammatory diet, we frequently concentrate on foods and supplements that reduce inflammation, boost the immune system, and promote overall health. However, there is another important aspect of health that is frequently overlooked: maintaining proper electrolyte balance. Electrolytes are essential for keeping your body running smoothly, and getting enough of them is key to feeling your best.

Electrolytes are minerals with an electric charge that are required for a variety of bodily functions. These are sodium, potassium, magnesium, calcium, chloride, and phosphate. While you might think that electrolytes are only important when you're sweating from intense exercise or heat, the truth is that they're essential for your body every day, even when you're just going about your normal routine.

Here's why electrolytes are important:

1. Fluid Balance and Hydration

Electrolytes help to regulate the balance of fluids inside and outside your cells, ensuring proper hydration. Dehydration is a common problem when following an anti-inflammatory diet, especially if you're focusing on eating more whole foods and limiting processed foods. If you don't keep your balance, you may feel sluggish, fatigued, or even get headaches.

2: Muscle Function

Electrolytes play an important role in muscle contraction. Muscle cramps, spasms, and weakness may result from a lack of potassium, calcium, and magnesium. This is especially true if you're increasing your activity levels or engaging in a lot of physical movement to improve your health in addition to diet changes.

3. Nervous Function

Your nerves rely on electrolytes to send and receive electrical signals between the brain and the body. Low electrolyte levels can interfere with your nervous system, causing symptoms such as dizziness, fatigue, and even mental fog.

4. Supporting Heart Health

Magnesium and potassium are essential for maintaining cardiac rhythm. If you don't get enough of these minerals, you're more likely to develop arrhythmias or irregular heartbeats. A well-balanced electrolyte intake promotes heart health and circulation.

5. Manage Inflammation

Electrolytes do not directly reduce inflammation, but they can help manage it. When you're properly hydrated and have balanced electrolytes, your body is better able to repair tissue, maintain healthy blood pressure, and support efficient nutrient absorption—all of which can have a positive impact on your inflammatory response.

If you're focusing on reducing inflammation in your body with an anti-inflammatory diet, you should also ensure that your electrolytes are in balance. This promotes your body's healing processes and overall health.

Top Sources of Natural Electrolytes

Instead of relying on processed sports drinks or synthetic electrolyte powders, it is always preferable to get your electrolytes from natural, whole foods. Many foods that are already staples in an anti-inflammatory diet—such as fruits, vegetables, nuts, and seeds—are high in electrolytes. Let's take a look at some of the best natural electrolyte sources that you should incorporate into your daily diet.

1. Coconut Water

Coconut water is an excellent natural source of electrolytes, particularly potassium. It's dubbed "nature's sports drink" for good reason: it's hydrating, low in sugar, and high in potassium, sodium, magnesium, and calcium. It's ideal for replenishing electrolytes after exercise or as a hydrating beverage all day.

- How to Use: Drink coconut water on its own, mix it into smoothies, or incorporate it into your cooking (e.g., rice or stews) for added flavor and nutrition.

2. Leafy greens (such as spinach, kale, and Swiss chard)
Leafy greens are high in magnesium and potassium, both of which are essential for hydration and muscle function. Kale and spinach, in particular, are nutrient dense and easy to incorporate into meals.

- How to Use: Mix spinach or kale into smoothies, salads, soups, or stir-fries. You can also make a quick and nutritious side dish by sautéing garlic and olive oil together.

3) Bananas
Bananas are famously high in potassium, one of the most important electrolytes for hydration and heart function. They're a great snack to have on the go.

- How to Use: Bananas can be eaten on their own or mixed into smoothies, yogurt bowls, or oatmeal. You can also freeze them to create a creamy base for dairy-free ice cream.

4) Avocados
Avocados are high in healthy fats, but they also contain plenty of potassium. They have a creamy texture and can be added to meals to increase electrolyte intake while providing a good source of healthy fat.

- How to Use: Mash avocado on whole grain toast, mix it into salads, top tacos or soups, or blend it into smoothies for a creamy texture.

5) Sweet Potatoes
Sweet potatoes are high in potassium and magnesium, which regulate fluid levels and support muscle and nerve function. They also contain a lot of fiber and antioxidants, making them ideal for an anti-inflammatory diet.

- How to Use: Roast or bake sweet potatoes as a side dish, mash them for a comforting alternative to mashed potatoes, or blend them into smoothies for a nutritional boost.

6. Yogurt and Kefir
Both yogurt and kefir are high in calcium and potassium, which are essential electrolytes for bone health and muscle function. Kefir, a fermented dairy drink, is high in probiotics, which can help with gut health and reduce inflammation.

- How to Use: Yogurt and kefir can be enjoyed as snacks or used as a base for smoothies. You can also mix them into oatmeal or create a yogurt parfait with fresh berries and nuts.

Sue Slaughter

7. Nuts and Seeds (including almonds, pumpkin seeds, and chia seeds)
Nuts and seeds contain high levels of magnesium, calcium, and potassium. Almonds, in particular, are high in magnesium, whereas pumpkin seeds contain both magnesium and zinc. Chia seeds are another great source of magnesium that can be easily added to your meals.

- How to Use: Snack on a handful of almonds or pumpkin seeds, sprinkle chia seeds on smoothies, salads, or yogurt, or blend them into your smoothie for added crunch.

8. Watermelon
Watermelon is a great hydrating fruit with plenty of potassium and magnesium. It also contains a lot of water, which keeps you hydrated and replenishes your electrolytes.

- How to Use: Watermelon can be consumed on its own or blended into a refreshing smoothie. It also makes an excellent addition to salads and fruit salads.

9) Sea Salt
While sodium is the most well-known electrolyte, it's important to note that too much sodium from processed foods can lead to high blood pressure and inflammation. However, a small amount of natural sea salt can help maintain electrolyte balance without overdoing it.

- How to Use: Use sea salt sparingly in cooking or sprinkle it on your dishes for a boost of flavor and electrolytes.

Developing a Daily Routine to Promote Electrolyte Intake

Now that you've learned about the best sources of natural electrolytes, let's look at how to incorporate them into your daily routine. The goal is to maintain a consistent, balanced electrolyte intake throughout the day, especially if you're on an anti-inflammatory diet.

Here's a simple daily routine that can help you maintain appropriate electrolyte levels:

1. Start the Day with Hydration
Begin your morning with a glass of electrolyte-infused water. To boost your hydration, start your morning routine with a pinch of sea salt or a splash of coconut water. Drinking water first thing in the morning also helps to kickstart your metabolism and aids in the detoxification process.

2. Have an electrolyte-rich breakfast
For breakfast, try a smoothie with spinach (magnesium), banana (potassium), avocado (healthy fats, potassium), and coconut water (electrolytes). For a more substantial breakfast, try a yogurt bowl topped with chia seeds, berries, and a sprinkle of nuts.

3. Consume Balanced, Electrolyte-Rich Meals
For lunch and dinner, include leafy greens (magnesium and calcium), sweet potatoes (potassium), lean proteins (chicken, fish, beans), and healthy fats (olive oil, avocado). To increase your mineral intake, serve with roasted vegetables or a salad.

4. Snack wisely
Between meals, choose electrolyte-rich snacks. A handful of almonds, pumpkin seeds, or some watermelon are excellent options. You can also drink a small amount of coconut water or kefir.

5. Stay Hydrated Throughout the Day
Drinking water throughout the day is essential, but you can also get more electrolytes by drinking coconut water or an electrolyte-enhanced drink (just make sure it's natural and free of artificial additives).

6. Finish Your Day With Magnesium
Magnesium is an electrolyte that promotes muscle relaxation and a good night's sleep. Consider including a small serving of magnesium-rich foods such as almonds or leafy greens in your evening meal, or drink a soothing cup of chamomile tea.

5: The Anti-Inflammatory Powerhouse

Certain anti-inflammatory ingredients stand out as true powerhouses. These foods are more than just healthy; they contain compounds that help reduce inflammation, boost your immune system, and promote overall wellness. Turmeric, ginger, and olive oil are among the top contenders in this category. Let's take a closer look at why they're so effective, how to incorporate them into your meals, and how to maximize their healing benefits.

1. Turmeric, the Golden Spice

Turmeric has long been used in traditional medicine, most notably in Ayurvedic and Chinese practices. Turmeric's active compound, curcumin, is responsible for its vibrant yellow color as well as its potent anti-inflammatory properties. Curcumin is well-known for its potent anti-inflammatory properties, and it has been extensively researched for its ability to regulate the body's inflammatory response.

According to research, curcumin can help reduce pro-inflammatory cytokines and enzymes in the body. It can also help reduce oxidative stress, which is another important factor in chronic inflammation. Turmeric is a must-have in your anti-inflammatory toolkit, whether you're suffering from joint pain, digestive issues, or simply want to protect yourself from long-term inflammation.

Health Benefits of Turmeric:
- Reduces joint pain and stiffness (effective for arthritis).
- Helps to regulate blood sugar levels and reduce insulin resistance.
- Promotes digestive health and relieves bloating or discomfort.
- May enhance cognitive function and lower the risk of Alzheimer's disease.
- Serves as a potent antioxidant, protecting cells from damage.

2. Ginger, the Zesty Healer

Ginger, like turmeric, has been used as medicine for centuries. It is well-known for its ability to soothe upset stomachs, as well as its potent anti-inflammatory and antioxidant properties. The active compound gingerol in ginger has been shown to inhibit the production of inflammatory compounds, and it works similarly to turmeric by lowering oxidative stress in the body.

Ginger is especially beneficial for digestive inflammation, making it an excellent supplement for people suffering from gut issues, bloating, or nausea. It has also been studied for its ability to reduce muscle soreness, making it an effective post-workout treatment for inflammation.

Health Benefits of Ginger:
- Reduces inflammation and pain in joints and muscles.
- Relieves digestive symptoms like nausea, bloating, and indigestion.
- May alleviate the severity of migraines and headaches.
- Promotes heart health by lowering cholesterol and improving circulation. - Naturally boosts immunity.

3. Olive Oil, the Heart-Healthy Fat

Olive oil is a staple of the Mediterranean diet, and for good reason: it's not only delicious but also high in healthy fats, which help reduce inflammation. The primary anti-inflammatory compound in olive oil is oleocanthal, which works similarly to ibuprofen in the body by inhibiting inflammatory pathways. Olive oil also contains polyphenols, which are antioxidants that help to reduce oxidative damage and inflammation.

Incorporating high-quality olive oil into your diet can help with heart health, brain function, and even longevity. It is a necessary fat for any anti-inflammatory diet plan.

Health Benefits of Olive Oil:
- Improves heart health by lowering LDL cholesterol and blood pressure.
- Has anti-inflammatory properties, which reduce the risk of chronic diseases such as diabetes, cancer, and arthritis.
- Supports healthy brain function and lowers the risk of cognitive decline.
- Promotes skin health by supplying essential fatty acids and antioxidants.

- Promotes the absorption of fat-soluble vitamins (such as vitamins A, D, E, and K).

Cooking with These Powerhouses to Maximize Their Health Benefits

Now that you understand why turmeric, ginger, and olive oil are so beneficial, let's look at how to cook with them to maximize their anti-inflammatory properties. The key is to use them in ways that preserve their nutrients while also allowing your body to absorb their healing properties.

1. How to Cook with Turmeric

Turmeric is extremely versatile in the kitchen and goes well with a wide range of savory dishes. Curcumin, on the other hand, is fat-soluble, which means that when combined with healthy fats, the body absorbs it more efficiently. That's why it pairs well with olive oil, coconut oil, and avocado.

Tips for Cooking with Turmeric:
- Pair it with black pepper**: Black pepper contains piperine, which enhances curcumin absorption in the body. Adding a pinch of black pepper to your turmeric dishes will boost their anti-inflammatory properties.
- Try it in warm dishes: Turmeric's beneficial compounds are released when heated, so it works best in warm dishes like soups, curries, and stews.
- Make turmeric tea: To make a soothing anti-inflammatory drink, combine turmeric with hot water, a pinch of black pepper, and a splash of honey or lemon. Add a teaspoon of coconut or olive oil for extra benefits.

2. Cooking With Ginger

Ginger can be used fresh or ground in cooking. It's ideal for adding a little zing to your meals and works well in both sweet and savory recipes. When using fresh ginger, peel it first, then slice or grate it according to how strong you want the flavor.

Tips for Cooking with Ginger:
- Incorporate fresh ginger into smoothies: Adding fresh ginger to your morning smoothie is an easy way to reap anti-inflammatory benefits. It pairs well with fruits such as pineapple, mango, and strawberries.
- Use it in stir-fries and soups: Ginger adds a zesty flavor to stir-fries and soups, and it pairs especially well with Asian-inspired dishes like stir-fried vegetables or chicken pho.
- Make ginger tea: Ginger tea is an excellent way to improve digestion and reduce inflammation. Simply slice fresh ginger and steep it in hot water with some honey and lemon.

3. Cooking in Olive Oil

Olive oil works best as a finishing oil or for cooking over low to medium heat. High heat can degrade the delicate antioxidants in olive oil, so avoid using it for frying. Instead, try incorporating it into your meals by drizzling it over cooked vegetables, adding it to dressings, or sautéing vegetables over medium heat.

How to Cook with Olive Oil:
- Use extra virgin olive oil. Extra virgin olive oil is the highest quality and contains the most antioxidants. It is minimally processed, preserving more of its health benefits.
- Prepare an olive oil dressing: Make a simple anti-inflammatory salad dressing by combining olive oil, balsamic vinegar, lemon juice, and your favorite herbs.
- Drizzle it on roasted vegetables: Drizzle olive oil over vegetables like sweet potatoes, Brussels sprouts, and cauliflower before roasting to help preserve their flavors and health benefits

SMOOTHIES AND BREAKFAST

Berry Turmeric Smoothie

Prep Time: 5 minutes

Total Time: 5 minutes

Servings: 1 large smoothie or 2 small

Ingredients:

1 cup mixed berries (blueberries, strawberries, or a combination)

1 small banana

1 tablespoon ground flaxseed

½ teaspoon turmeric

Pinch of black pepper

1 cup coconut milk

½ cup spinach

1. If you're using frozen berries, no need to thaw them—this will make your smoothie even colder and more refreshing! Peel the banana and add it to your blender. Wash the spinach thoroughly to remove any dirt or grit.

2. In your blender, combine the mixed berries, banana, ground flaxseed, turmeric, black pepper, coconut milk, and spinach. Blend on high until smooth and creamy. If the smoothie is too thick for your liking, you can add a little more coconut milk to reach your desired consistency.

3. Give it a quick taste. If you prefer a slightly sweeter smoothie, you can add a touch of honey, maple syrup, or a couple of extra berries. If you'd like a more pronounced turmeric flavor, feel free to add a little extra turmeric.

4. Pour into a glass or a to-go container for a delicious breakfast or snack. Top with a few more flaxseeds or a sprinkle of cinnamon if you like.

Green Smoothie

Prep Time: 5 minutes

Serving Size: 1 large smoothie
(about 16-18 oz)

Ingredients:

1 cup kale or spinach

½ avocado

½ cucumber

½ green apple

1 tablespoon fresh ginger (grated)

Juice of ½ lemon

1 cup coconut water

1. If using kale, remove the tough stems. Peel the avocado and scoop out the flesh. Peel the cucumber (optional) and slice it into smaller pieces. Core the green apple and cut it into chunks. Grate the fresh ginger and squeeze the juice of the lemon.

2. In a blender, combine the kale (or spinach), avocado, cucumber, green apple, ginger, lemon juice, and coconut water. Blend until smooth and creamy.

3. If the smoothie is too thick, you can add a little more coconut water or a few ice cubes to reach your desired consistency.

Cherry Ginger Smoothie

Prep Time: 5 minutes

Serving Size: 1 large smoothie
(about 16-18 oz)

Ingredients:

1 cup frozen cherries

½ cup pineapple chunks

1 tablespoon fresh ginger (grated)

1 teaspoon ground flaxseed

1 cup coconut or almond milk

1. Peel and grate the fresh ginger. If you're using unsweetened coconut or almond milk, ensure it's the variety with no added sugars.

2. In a blender, combine the frozen cherries, pineapple chunks, grated ginger, ground flaxseed, and coconut or almond milk. Blend on high until smooth and creamy.

3. If the smoothie is too thick, feel free to add a bit more coconut or almond milk to reach your desired texture.

Tropical Turmeric Smoothie

Prep Time: 5 minutes

Serving Size: 1 large smoothie (about 16-18 oz)

Ingredients:

½ cup mango chunks

½ cup pineapple

½ banana

½ teaspoon turmeric

Pinch of black pepper

1 cup coconut milk

1. If you're using fresh mango and pineapple, cut them into chunks. Peel the banana and add it to the blender.

2. In a blender, combine the mango, pineapple, banana, turmeric, black pepper, and coconut milk. Blend until smooth and creamy.

3. If the smoothie is too thick, you can add a little more coconut milk to reach your desired consistency.

Avocado Mint Smoothie

Prep Time: 5 minutes

Serving Size: 1 large smoothie
(about 16-18 oz)

Ingredients:

½ avocado

½ cup cucumber (peeled, if
preferred)

Small handful of fresh mint
leaves

Juice of ½ lime

1 cup coconut water

1 tablespoon hemp seeds

1. Peel and pit the avocado. Slice the cucumber into smaller chunks. Squeeze the juice from half a lime. Rinse the fresh mint leaves.

2. In a blender, combine the avocado, cucumber, mint leaves, lime juice, coconut water, and hemp seeds. Blend until smooth and creamy.

3. If the smoothie is too thick, add a little more coconut water to thin it out to your desired texture.

4. Pour into a glass, garnish with extra mint leaves if desired

Carrot Cake Smoothie

Prep Time: 5 minutes

Serving Size: 1 large smoothie
(about 16-18 oz)

Ingredients:

1 small carrot, grated

½ banana

1 tablespoon shredded coconut

¼ teaspoon cinnamon

¼ teaspoon vanilla extract

1 tablespoon walnuts

1 cup coconut milk

1. Peel and grate the carrot. Slice the banana and break the walnuts into smaller pieces if needed.

2. In a blender, combine the grated carrot, banana, shredded coconut, cinnamon, vanilla extract, walnuts, and coconut milk. Blend until smooth and creamy.

3. If the smoothie is too thick, you can add a bit more coconut milk or a splash of water to reach your desired consistency.

Sue Slaughter

Fig and Blackberry Smoothie

Prep Time: 5 minutes

Serving Size: 1 large smoothie
(about 16-18 oz)

Ingredients:

3 fresh or dried figs (soaked if dried)

½ cup blackberries

½ banana

1 tablespoon chia seeds

1 cup coconut or almond milk

1. If using dried figs, soak them in warm water for 10-15 minutes to soften. Once softened, remove the stems. Slice the banana, rinse the blackberries, and measure out the chia seeds.

2. In a blender, combine the soaked figs (or fresh figs), blackberries, banana, chia seeds, and coconut or almond milk. Blend until smooth and creamy.

3. If the smoothie is too thick, add a little more coconut or almond milk to thin it out to your desired consistency.

Sweet Potato Pie Smoothie

Prep Time: 5 minutes

Cooking Time: 10-15 minutes (if cooking the sweet potato)

Serving Size: 1 large smoothie (about 16-18 oz)

Ingredients:

½ cup cooked sweet potato

½ banana

1 date, pitted

¼ teaspoon cinnamon

Pinch of nutmeg

1 cup coconut milk

1. If you haven't already, cook the sweet potato until soft (you can bake, steam, or microwave it). Peel the banana and pit the date.

2. In a blender, combine the cooked sweet potato, banana, date, cinnamon, nutmeg, and coconut milk. Blend until smooth and creamy.

3. If the smoothie is too thick, you can add a little more coconut milk or water to thin it out.

Turmeric Chia Pudding

Prep Time: 5 minutes

Refrigeration Time: 4 hours or overnight

Serving Size: 1 serving (about 1 cup)

Ingredients:

3 tablespoons chia seeds

1 cup coconut milk

½ teaspoon turmeric

Pinch of black pepper

1 teaspoon honey

Topped with berries and coconut flakes

1. In a bowl or jar, mix together the chia seeds, coconut milk, turmeric, black pepper, and honey (if using). Stir well to ensure that the turmeric is evenly distributed.

2. Cover the bowl or jar and refrigerate for at least 4 hours or overnight. The chia seeds will absorb the coconut milk, creating a thick, pudding-like consistency.

3. Once the chia pudding has set, give it a good stir. Top with fresh berries (such as blueberries, strawberries, or raspberries) and a sprinkle of coconut flakes.

Salmon and Avocado Bowl

Prep Time: 5 minutes

Serving Size: 1 serving

Ingredients:

3 oz wild-caught smoked salmon

½ avocado, sliced

Handful of arugula

Squeeze of lemon juice

1 tablespoon olive oil

Fresh herbs (dill or parsley)

1. In a bowl, place a handful of fresh arugula as the base. Arrange the smoked salmon on top, then add the sliced avocado.

2. Drizzle olive oil over the top and squeeze fresh lemon juice to add brightness.

3. Sprinkle with fresh herbs like dill or parsley for a burst of flavor and color.

Sweet Potato Breakfast Hash

Prep Time: 5 minutes

Cooking Time: 25 minutes

Serving Size: 1

Ingredients:

1 small sweet potato, diced and roasted

¼ cup sautéed kale

¼ onion, diced

¼ bell pepper, diced

½ avocado, sliced

Fresh herbs (such as parsley or cilantro)

Olive oil for cooking

1. Preheat your oven to 400°F (200°C). Toss the diced sweet potato in a bit of olive oil and spread it on a baking sheet. Roast for 20-25 minutes or until the sweet potato is tender and lightly browned, stirring halfway through.

2. While the sweet potato is roasting, heat a small amount of olive oil in a pan over medium heat. Add the diced onion and bell pepper, and sauté for 4-5 minutes, until softened. Add the kale and cook for another 2-3 minutes until wilted.

3. Once the sweet potatoes are done roasting, add them to the pan with the sautéed vegetables and mix gently.

4. Top the hash with sliced avocado and sprinkle fresh herbs over the top. Serve

Coconut Yogurt Parfait

Prep Time: 5 minutes

Serving Size: 1

Ingredients:

1 cup coconut yogurt

¼ cup blueberries

1 tablespoon pumpkin seeds

1 tablespoon ground flaxseed

1 teaspoon honey

1. In a bowl or glass, spoon in the coconut yogurt as the first layer.

2. Layer the blueberries on top of the yogurt. Then sprinkle the pumpkin seeds and ground flaxseed over the blueberries.

3. If you prefer a sweeter parfait, drizzle a teaspoon of honey on top.

Breakfast Bowl

Prep Time: 5 minutes (if quinoa is already cooked)

Cooking Time: 15 minutes (for quinoa)

Serving Size: 1

Ingredients:

½ cup cooked quinoa

½ cup mixed berries

1 tablespoon walnuts, chopped

1 tablespoon pumpkin seeds

1 teaspoon cinnamon

Coconut milk to moisten

1. If you haven't already, cook the quinoa according to package instructions. Typically, this involves rinsing it and simmering in water for about 15 minutes until the liquid is absorbed.

2. In a bowl, add the cooked quinoa as the base. Top with mixed berries, walnuts, and pumpkin seeds.

3. Sprinkle the cinnamon evenly over the bowl for an added anti-inflammatory boost and flavor.

4. Drizzle coconut milk over the top to moisten the quinoa and create a creamy texture.

5. Stir everything together

Breakfast Porridge

Prep Time: 5 minutes

Cooking Time: 20-25 minutes

Serving Size: 1

Ingredients:

½ cup gluten-free steel cut oats

1 cup bone broth (chicken, beef, or vegetable)

1 tablespoon olive oil

¼ avocado, sliced

Fresh herbs (such as parsley, chives, or cilantro)

Turmeric and black pepper (to taste)

1. In a medium pot, bring the bone broth to a boil. Add the steel cut oats, reduce the heat, and simmer uncovered for about 20-25 minutes, or until the oats are soft and have absorbed the broth.

2. Once the oats are cooked, stir in the turmeric and black pepper to taste. Add the olive oil for a creamy, rich texture.

3. Spoon the porridge into a bowl, and top with sliced avocado and fresh herbs of your choice for a burst of flavor and freshness.

Sautéed Greens with Poached Eggs

Prep Time: 5 minutes

Cooking Time: 5-7 minutes

Serving Size: 1

Ingredients:

2 cups sautéed spinach or kale

2 poached eggs

1 tablespoon olive oil

1 clove garlic, minced

Lemon juice (to taste)

Fresh herbs (such as parsley, dill, or basil)

1. Heat the olive oil in a pan over medium heat. Add the minced garlic and sauté for about 1 minute, until fragrant. Add the spinach or kale and cook for 3-4 minutes, stirring occasionally, until the greens are wilted and tender. Season with salt and pepper to taste.

2. While the greens are cooking, poach the eggs in a separate pot. To do this, bring a pot of water to a gentle simmer and add a splash of vinegar. Crack each egg into a small bowl and gently slide it into the water. Cook for about 3-4 minutes until the whites are set but the yolks are still runny. Remove with a slotted spoon.

3. Plate the sautéed greens and top with the poached eggs. Drizzle a bit of lemon juice over the top for brightness and sprinkle with fresh herbs for extra flavor.

Butternut Squash Bowl

Prep Time: 5 minutes

Cooking Time: 25 minutes

Serving Size: 1

Ingredients:

1 cup roasted butternut squash (diced)

2 tablespoons pumpkin seeds

1 tablespoon coconut oil

Cinnamon and nutmeg (to taste)

2 tablespoons coconut flakes

1. Preheat your oven to 400°F (200°C). Toss the diced butternut squash with a little olive oil, salt, and pepper. Spread it in a single layer on a baking sheet and roast for 20-25 minutes, or until tender and slightly caramelized, stirring halfway through.

2. Once the squash is roasted, place it in a bowl. Drizzle with coconut oil, and sprinkle with cinnamon and nutmeg to taste. Toss gently to combine.

3. Add the pumpkin seeds and coconut flakes on top of the butternut squash.

Sue Slaughter

Sardine and Cucumber Toast

Prep Time: 5 minutes

Serving Size: 1

Ingredients:

1 slice gluten-free bread

Wild-caught sardines (about 2-3 sardines, drained)

¼ avocado, mashed

Cucumber slices

Lemon juice (to taste)

Fresh herbs (such as parsley or dill)

1. Lightly toast the gluten-free bread until golden and crisp.

2. In a small bowl, mash the avocado with a fork and spread it evenly over the toasted bread.

3. Place the sardines on top of the mashed avocado, followed by a layer of cucumber slices.

4. Squeeze fresh lemon juice over the toast and sprinkle with fresh herbs for extra flavor.

Sweet Potato Boats

Prep Time: 5 minutes

Cooking Time: 40-45 minutes

Serving Size: 1 (1 sweet potato split into 2 boats)

Ingredients:

1 baked sweet potato

2 tablespoons almond butter

Sprinkle of cinnamon

1 tablespoon coconut flakes

1 teaspoon honey

1. Preheat your oven to 400°F (200°C). Pierce the sweet potato with a fork a few times and place it on a baking sheet. Bake for 40-45 minutes, or until tender when pierced with a fork. Let it cool slightly before handling.

2. Slice the baked sweet potato lengthwise to create two "boats." Gently scoop out a little of the flesh to create room for the toppings.

3. Spread 1 tablespoon of almond butter into each sweet potato boat. Sprinkle with cinnamon, then add coconut flakes and drizzle with honey (if using).

Sue Slaughter

Berry and Coconut Bowl

Prep Time: 5 minutes

Serving Size: 1

Ingredients:

½ cup mixed berries (blueberries, strawberries, raspberries, etc.)

¼ cup shredded coconut

2 tablespoons pumpkin seeds

2 tablespoons hemp seeds

Coconut yogurt or coconut milk (to moisten)

1. In a bowl, place the mixed berries as the base of the bowl.

2. Sprinkle the shredded coconut, pumpkin seeds, and hemp seeds over the berries.

3. Drizzle coconut yogurt or milk over the top to create a creamy texture.

4. Stir everything together

Herbal Congee

Prep Time: 5 minutes

Cooking Time: 20 minutes

Serving Size: 1

Ingredients:

½ cup white rice, cooked in 2 cups water

1 tablespoon fresh ginger, grated

1 tablespoon fresh turmeric, grated

2 cups bone broth (chicken, beef, or vegetable)

Cilantro, for garnish

Green onions, for garnish

Drizzle of olive oil

1. In a medium saucepan, cook the rice according to package instructions using 2 cups of water. Once cooked, set it aside.

2. In the same saucepan, add the bone broth, grated ginger, and grated turmeric. Bring to a gentle simmer and cook for 5-10 minutes to allow the flavors to infuse.

3. Add the cooked rice to the pot with the broth, ginger, and turmeric. Stir well to combine and let it simmer for another 5-10 minutes until the rice has absorbed some of the liquid and becomes a thick, porridge-like consistency.

4. Serve the congee in a bowl and drizzle with olive oil. Top with fresh cilantro and green onions for extra flavor.

Sue Slaughter

SALADS AND SMALL BITES

Wild Salmon and Avocado Salad

Prep Time: 10 minutes

Cooking Time: 10 minutes (for grilling the salmon)

Serving Size: 1

Ingredients:

Mixed greens (arugula, spinach)

1 grilled wild-caught salmon fillet

½ avocado, sliced

½ cucumber, sliced

¼ red onion (soaked in water to reduce harshness)

Fresh herbs (dill, parsley)

Dressing:

1 tablespoon olive oil

1 tablespoon lemon juice

½ teaspoon turmeric

Salt and pepper to taste

1. Preheat a grill or grill pan over medium heat. Season the salmon fillet with salt and pepper, then grill for about 4-5 minutes on each side, or until the fish flakes easily with a fork. Set aside to cool slightly before flaking into large pieces.

2. In a large bowl, combine the mixed greens, sliced avocado, cucumber, and soaked red onion.

3. In a small bowl, whisk together olive oil, lemon juice, turmeric, salt, and pepper until well combined.

4. Add the grilled salmon pieces to the salad. Drizzle the dressing over the top and toss gently to combine.

5. Sprinkle fresh dill and parsley over the salad for added flavor and freshness.

Sue Slaughter

Tropical Kale and Mango Salad

Prep Time: 10 minutes

Cooking Time: 5 minutes (for toasting coconut)

Serving Size: 2 servings

Ingredients:

For the Salad:

2 cups kale, chopped and massaged with olive oil

1 fresh mango, peeled and chopped into chunks

¼ cup toasted coconut flakes

2 tablespoons sliced almonds

2 tablespoons fresh cilantro, chopped

For the Dressing:

Juice of 1 lime

1 teaspoon honey

1 teaspoon freshly grated ginger

2 tablespoons olive oil

1. In a large bowl, drizzle olive oil over the chopped kale. Use your hands to gently massage the kale for about 2-3 minutes, until it softens and darkens in color. This step helps to break down the tough fibers and makes the kale more tender.

2. In a small skillet over medium heat, toast the coconut flakes for 2-3 minutes, stirring frequently until golden and fragrant. Remove from heat and set aside.

3. In a small bowl, whisk together the lime juice, honey, grated ginger, and olive oil until well combined.

4. Add the fresh mango chunks, toasted coconut flakes, sliced almonds, and chopped cilantro to the massaged kale.

5. Drizzle the lime and ginger dressing over the salad and toss gently to combine.

Roasted Root Vegetable Salad

Prep Time: 10 minutes

Cooking Time: 30 minutes

Serving Size: 2-3 servings

Ingredients:

Mixed greens (such as spinach, arugula, or baby kale)

1 small sweet potato, peeled and diced

1 small beet, peeled and diced

2 medium carrots, peeled and sliced

2 tablespoons walnuts, toasted

Fresh thyme

For the Dressing**:

2 tablespoons apple cider vinegar

3 tablespoons olive oil

1 teaspoon fresh or dried herbs (such as thyme, oregano, or rosemary)

Salt and pepper to taste

1. Preheat your oven to 400°F (200°C). Arrange the diced sweet potato, beet, and carrot on a baking sheet in a single layer. Drizzle with a little olive oil, salt, and pepper, and toss to coat. Roast for 25-30 minutes, or until tender and slightly caramelized, stirring halfway through.

2. While the vegetables are roasting, toast the walnuts in a small pan over medium heat for 3-4 minutes, until fragrant and golden brown. Set aside to cool.

3. In a small bowl, whisk together the apple cider vinegar, olive oil, herbs, salt, and pepper until well combined.

4. In a large bowl, toss the mixed greens with the roasted vegetables. Drizzle the dressing over the top and toss to combine.

5. Top the salad with the toasted walnuts and fresh thyme.

Wild Blueberry Spinach Salad

Prep Time: 10 minutes

Cooking Time: 3 minutes (for toasting pumpkin seeds)

Serving Size: 1-2 servings

Ingredients:

2 cups baby spinach

½ cup fresh blueberries

½ small fennel bulb, thinly sliced

2 tablespoons toasted pumpkin seeds

For the Dressing**:

1 tablespoon olive oil

1 tablespoon lemon juice

1 teaspoon honey

Fresh herbs (such as parsley or dill)

Salt and pepper, to taste

1. In a large bowl, toss together the baby spinach, fresh blueberries, and thinly sliced fennel.

2. In a dry skillet, toast the pumpkin seeds over medium heat for 2-3 minutes, until lightly browned and fragrant. Set aside to cool.

3. In a small bowl, whisk together the olive oil, lemon juice, honey (if using), fresh herbs, salt, and pepper until well combined.

4. Drizzle the dressing over the salad and toss gently to coat. Top with the toasted pumpkin seeds.

Mediterranean Herb Salad

Prep Time: 10 minutes

Serving Size: 2 servings

Ingredients:

Mixed greens (such as arugula, spinach, and romaine)

1 cucumber, thinly sliced

½ cup olives (such as Kalamata or green olives), pitted and sliced

¼ red onion, thinly sliced

Fresh herbs: 1 tablespoon chopped mint, parsley, and oregano

Dressing:

2 tablespoons olive oil

1 tablespoon lemon juice

1 clove garlic, minced

1. In a large bowl, combine the mixed greens, cucumber slices, olives, red onion, and fresh herbs.

2. In a small bowl, whisk together the olive oil, lemon juice, and minced garlic. Season with salt and pepper to taste.

3. Pour the dressing over the salad and toss gently to combine, ensuring all the ingredients are evenly coated.

Sweet Potato Avocado Bites

Prep Time: 5 minutes

Cooking Time: 20-25 minutes

Serving Size: 1 (about 6-8 bites depending on size of sweet potato)

Ingredients:

Roasted sweet potato rounds (about 1 small sweet potato)

½ avocado, mashed

Microgreens (such as arugula or sprouts)

Drizzle of olive oil

Squeeze of lemon juice

1. Preheat your oven to 400°F (200°C). Slice the sweet potato into ¼-inch thick rounds and arrange them on a baking sheet. Drizzle with olive oil, season with salt and pepper, and roast for 20-25 minutes, or until tender and slightly crispy on the edges.

2. While the sweet potato rounds are roasting, mash the avocado with a fork until creamy. Set aside.

3. Once the sweet potato rounds are done, top each round with a generous scoop of mashed avocado.

4. Add a few microgreens on top of each bite and drizzle with olive oil and a squeeze of lemon juice.

Turmeric Cauliflower Bites

Serves: 4

Prep Time: 10 minutes

Cooking Time: 30 minutes

Ingredients:

1 medium cauliflower, cut into florets

1 tablespoon olive oil

1 teaspoon turmeric powder

1/2 teaspoon ground ginger

2 cloves garlic, minced

Salt and pepper, to taste

1/4 cup toasted pine nuts

Fresh cilantro, chopped

1. Preheat your oven to 400°F (200°C).

2. In a large mixing bowl, toss the cauliflower florets with olive oil, turmeric, ginger, minced garlic, salt, and pepper until evenly coated.

3. Spread the seasoned cauliflower florets in a single layer on a baking sheet. Roast in the preheated oven for 25-30 minutes, or until the cauliflower is tender and slightly crispy on the edges, flipping halfway through.

4. While the cauliflower is roasting, toast the pine nuts in a dry pan over medium heat for 2-3 minutes, stirring occasionally, until they are golden brown. Remove from heat and set aside.

5. Once the cauliflower bites are done roasting, remove them from the oven. Sprinkle with the toasted pine nuts and fresh cilantro before serving.

Cucumber Sushi Rolls

Prep Time: 10 minutes

Servings: 2

Ingredients:

1 large cucumber, thinly sliced lengthwise

½ avocado, mashed

1 small carrot, julienned

3 oz wild-caught salmon or tuna, cooked or raw (sushi-grade)

¼ cup sprouts (e.g., alfalfa or broccoli)

1 tbsp coconut aminos

1. Using a vegetable peeler or mandoline, slice the cucumber lengthwise into thin, even strips. Pat dry with a paper towel to remove excess moisture.

2. In a small bowl, mash the avocado with a fork until smooth.

3. Lay out a cucumber strip, spread a thin layer of mashed avocado over it, then place a few pieces of carrot, salmon/tuna, and sprouts at one end.

4. Gently roll up the cucumber strip, securing it with a toothpick if necessary. Repeat with the remaining ingredients.

5. Arrange the rolls on a plate and serve with coconut aminos for dipping.

Zucchini Herb Fritters with Coconut Yogurt

Prep Time: 10 minutes

Cook Time: 10 minutes

Servings: 2-3

Ingredients:

2 medium zucchinis, grated (about 2 cups, excess water squeezed out)

1 egg (or flax egg for AIP: 1 tbsp ground flaxseed + 3 tbsp water)

¼ cup coconut flour

2 tbsp fresh dill, chopped

2 tbsp fresh parsley, chopped

½ tsp sea salt

¼ tsp black pepper (omit for AIP)

2 tbsp olive oil

½ cup coconut yogurt

1. Grate the zucchinis and squeeze out excess water using a clean kitchen towel.

2. In a bowl, combine grated zucchini, egg, coconut flour, dill, parsley, salt, and pepper. Mix well until a thick batter forms.

3. Scoop small portions of the batter and form into patties.

4. Heat olive oil in a skillet over medium heat. Cook the fritters for about 3-4 minutes per side, until golden brown and crispy.

5. Plate the fritters and serve with coconut yogurt on the side.

Stuffed Mushroom Caps with Spinach

Prep Time: 10 minutes

Cook Time: 15-18 minutes

Servings: 2

Ingredients:

4 large portobello mushroom caps, stems removed

2 cups fresh spinach, chopped

2 cloves garlic, minced

2 tbsp fresh herbs (parsley, thyme, or basil), chopped

2 tbsp olive oil, divided

¼ cup toasted pine nuts

½ tsp sea salt

¼ tsp black pepper (omit for AIP)

1. Preheat the oven to 375°F (190°C). Wipe the mushroom caps clean and remove stems. Place them on a baking sheet, gill-side up.

2. Heat 1 tbsp olive oil in a pan over medium heat. Add garlic and cook for 1 minute. Stir in spinach, herbs, salt, and pepper. Sauté until the spinach is wilted (about 2 minutes). Remove from heat.

3. Spoon the spinach mixture evenly into the mushroom caps. Drizzle with the remaining olive oil.

4. Place in the oven and bake for 15-18 minutes, until the mushrooms are tender.

5. Remove from the oven and sprinkle toasted pine nuts on top. Serve warm.

Soups, Stews and Sauces

Sue Slaughter

Prep Time: 10 minutes

Cook Time: 20-25 minutes

Servings: 4

Ingredients:

4 cups homemade bone broth (chicken or beef)

1 carrot, diced

1 celery stalk, diced

½ onion, chopped

1-inch piece fresh ginger, grated

1-inch piece fresh turmeric, grated (or ½ tsp ground turmeric)

2 cups leafy greens (kale or spinach), chopped

½ tsp sea salt (adjust to taste)

1 tbsp fresh herbs (parsley, thyme), chopped

Bone Broth Soup

1. In a large pot, heat a small amount of bone broth over medium heat. Add onion, carrot, and celery. Sauté for 3-4 minutes until softened.

2. Pour in the remaining bone broth. Stir in grated ginger, turmeric, and sea salt.

3. Bring to a gentle boil, then reduce heat and let simmer for 15-20 minutes.

4. Stir in the leafy greens and fresh herbs. Simmer for another 3-5 minutes until the greens are wilted.

5. Ladle into bowls

Prep Time: 10 minutes

Cook Time: 35-40 minutes

Servings: 4

Ingredients:

1 medium butternut squash, peeled, seeded, and cubed

1 tbsp olive oil (or coconut oil)

1 small onion, thinly sliced

2 cups bone broth (chicken or beef)

1 cup full-fat coconut milk

1 tbsp fresh sage, chopped

½ tsp cinnamon

¼ tsp nutmeg

½ tsp sea salt

Creamy Butternut Squash Soup

1. Preheat oven to 400°F (200°C). Toss the squash cubes with olive oil and spread them on a baking sheet. Roast for 25-30 minutes until soft and caramelized.

2. In a large pot, heat a bit of oil over medium heat. Add the onions and cook for 8-10 minutes until golden and soft.

3. Add the roasted squash, bone broth, cinnamon, nutmeg, sea salt, and sage. Simmer for 10 minutes to blend the flavors.

4. Use an immersion blender to puree the soup until creamy. Alternatively, transfer to a blender and blend in batches.

5. Pour in the coconut milk, stirring until smooth. Simmer for another 3 minutes, then remove from heat.

6. Ladle into bowls and garnish with extra sage or a sprinkle of cinnamon.

Wild Salmon Chowder

Prep Time: 10 minutes

Cook Time: 20 minutes

Servings: 4

Ingredients:

2 fillets (6 oz each) wild-caught salmon, skin removed and cut into chunks

1 tbsp olive oil or coconut oil

1 leek, white and light green parts, sliced

½ onion, chopped

1 celery stalk, diced

1 carrot, diced

2 cups cauliflower florets (replaces potatoes)

2 cups bone broth (chicken or fish)

1 cup coconut milk (full-fat, canned)

1 tbsp fresh dill, chopped

1 tsp fresh thyme leaves

½ tsp sea salt

¼ tsp black pepper (omit for AIP)

1. In a large pot, heat oil over medium heat. Add leeks, onions, celery, and carrots. Sauté for 3-4 minutes until softened.

2. Stir in cauliflower florets and bone broth. Bring to a gentle simmer and cook for 10 minutes until the cauliflower is tender.

3. Pour in the coconut milk, then add salmon chunks. Simmer for another 5-7 minutes until the salmon is fully cooked and flakes easily.

4. Stir in fresh dill, thyme, sea salt, and black pepper (if using). Let sit for a minute, then serve warm.

Chicken and Rice Soup

Prep Time: 10 minutes

Cook Time: 15-20 minutes

Servings: 4

Ingredients:

2 cups shredded organic chicken (cooked)

1½ cups cauliflower rice

1 carrot, diced

1 celery stalk, diced

½ onion, chopped

4 cups bone broth (chicken)

1 tsp fresh thyme, chopped

1 tsp fresh rosemary, chopped

1 tbsp fresh parsley, chopped

½ tsp sea salt

Zest of ½ lemon

1. In a large pot, heat a small amount of bone broth over medium heat. Add onion, carrot, and celery. Sauté for 3-4 minutes until softened.

2. Pour in the remaining bone broth and stir in thyme, rosemary, and sea salt. Bring to a simmer.

3. Stir in the shredded chicken and cauliflower rice. Simmer for 10-12 minutes until the cauliflower is tender.

4. Stir in lemon zest and fresh parsley before serving.

5. Ladle into bowls

Moroccan Lamb Stew

Prep Time: 15 minutes

Cook Time: 50 minutes

Servings: 4

Ingredients:

1 lb grass-fed lamb, cut into cubes

1 medium sweet potato, peeled and diced

2 carrots, sliced

1 small onion, chopped

2 cloves garlic, minced

1-inch piece fresh ginger, grated (or ½ tsp ground ginger)

1 tsp turmeric

½ tsp cinnamon

½ tsp sea salt

¼ tsp black pepper (omit for AIP)

2 cups bone broth (chicken or beef)

1 tbsp olive oil

2 tbsp fresh cilantro, chopped

1. Heat olive oil in a large pot over medium heat. Add lamb cubes and sear until browned on all sides (about 5 minutes). Remove and set aside.

2. In the same pot, add onion, garlic, and ginger. Sauté for 2-3 minutes until fragrant.

3. Stir in turmeric, cinnamon, salt, and pepper. Cook for 30 seconds to enhance the flavors.

4. Return the lamb to the pot. Add sweet potatoes, carrots, and bone broth. Bring to a boil, then reduce heat to low and let simmer for 45-50 minutes, until the lamb is tender.

5. Stir in fresh cilantro before serving.

Coconut Seafood Stew

Prep Time: 10 minutes

Cook Time: 15 minutes

Servings: 4

Ingredients:

½ lb wild-caught white fish (cod, halibut, or snapper), cut into chunks

½ lb shrimp, peeled and deveined

½ lb scallops

1 fennel bulb, thinly sliced

1 leek, white and light green parts, thinly sliced

1 carrot, diced

1 can (13.5 oz) full-fat coconut milk

2 cups seafood or vegetable broth

1 tbsp fresh lime juice

1 tbsp olive oil or coconut oil

1 tbsp fresh dill, chopped

1 tbsp fresh parsley, chopped

½ tsp sea salt

1. In a large pot, heat oil over medium heat. Add fennel, leeks, and carrots. Sauté for 5-7 minutes until softened.

2. Pour in the seafood or vegetable broth and coconut milk. Stir well and bring to a gentle simmer.

3. Add the white fish, shrimp, and scallops to the pot. Let simmer for 5-7 minutes, until the seafood is opaque and cooked through.

4. Stir in lime juice, dill, parsley, and sea salt. Let cook for another minute, then remove from heat.

5. Ladle into bowls

Sue Slaughter

Prep Time: 10 minutes

Cook Time: 25-30 minutes

Servings: 4

Ingredients:

1 lb ground organic turkey

1 medium zucchini, diced

1 large carrot, diced

1 cup mushrooms, sliced

1 leek, chopped (white and light green parts only)

2 cloves garlic, minced

4 cups bone broth (chicken or beef)

1 tsp fresh thyme, chopped

1 tsp fresh rosemary, chopped

½ tsp sea salt

1 tbsp olive oil

Turkey and Vegetable Stew

1. Heat olive oil in a large pot over medium heat. Add leeks and garlic, sautéing for 2-3 minutes until fragrant.

2. Add the ground turkey, breaking it up with a spoon. Cook until browned, about 5-7 minutes.

3. Stir in zucchini, carrots, and mushrooms. Cook for another 3 minutes.

4. Add bone broth, thyme, rosemary, and sea salt. Bring to a gentle boil.

5. Reduce heat to low and let the stew simmer for 20-25 minutes until vegetables are tender.

6. Ladle into bowls

Basil and Avocado Sauce

Prep Time: 5 minutes

Servings: 4 (2 tbsp per serving)

Ingredients:

2 ripe avocados, pitted and peeled

1 cup fresh basil leaves

2 tbsp olive oil

1 clove garlic, minced

2 tbsp lemon juice (freshly squeezed)

½ tsp sea salt

Water

1. In a blender or food processor, combine the avocados, fresh basil, olive oil, garlic, lemon juice, and sea salt.

2. Process until the mixture is smooth and creamy. If the sauce is too thick, add water, 1 tbsp at a time, until the desired consistency is reached.

3. Taste the sauce and add more salt or lemon juice, if needed, to balance the flavors.

4. Toss with zucchini noodles for a light pasta alternative or use as a dip for veggies or crackers.

Turmeric Sauce

Prep Time: 5 minutes

Cook Time: 10 minutes

Servings: 4 (2 tbsp per serving)

Ingredients:

1 cup coconut milk (full-fat or light)

1 tbsp fresh turmeric, grated (or 1 tsp ground turmeric)

1 tbsp fresh ginger, grated

2 cloves garlic, minced

1 tsp honey

1 tbsp lime juice (freshly squeezed)

2 tbsp fresh cilantro, chopped

1. Grate the fresh turmeric and ginger, and mince the garlic.

2. In a small saucepan, combine coconut milk, grated turmeric, ginger, and garlic. Stir and bring to a simmer over medium heat.

3. Let the mixture simmer for 5-7 minutes, stirring occasionally, until it thickens slightly.

4. Stir in the honey (if using) and lime juice, and cook for another minute.

5. Remove from heat and stir in fresh cilantro for added flavor and freshness.

6. Drizzle over seafood, roasted vegetables, or grains.

Herb Pesto (No Dairy)

Prep Time: 10 minutes

Servings: 6-8 (2 tbsp per serving)

Ingredients:

1 cup fresh basil leaves, packed

1 cup fresh parsley leaves, packed

2 tbsp olive oil

2 cloves garlic, minced

¼ cup toasted pine nuts or walnuts

2 tbsp nutritional yeast

1 tbsp fresh lemon juice

Sea salt, to taste

Freshly ground black pepper (omit for AIP)

1. In a food processor or blender, combine the basil, parsley, garlic, toasted pine nuts or walnuts, nutritional yeast, and lemon juice.

2. With the food processor running, slowly add olive oil until the mixture reaches a smooth, spreadable consistency.

3. Taste and add sea salt or more lemon juice, if desired. Blend again to combine.

4. Toss with zucchini noodles, drizzle over roasted proteins, or serve as a topping for vegetables.

Sue Slaughter

VEGETARIAN MAINS

Roasted Root Vegetable with Turmeric-Tahini Dressing

Prep Time: 10 minutes

Cook Time: 25-30 minutes

Servings: 2

Ingredients:

Base:

2 cups cauliflower rice

Toppings:

1 small sweet potato, peeled and cubed

1 beet, peeled and cubed

1 carrot, sliced

1 parsnip, sliced

1 tbsp olive oil

½ tsp sea salt

Protein:

2 tbsp pumpkin seeds

2 tbsp sunflower seeds

Turmeric-Tahini Dressing:

2 tbsp tahini

1 tbsp olive oil

1 tbsp lemon juice

½ tsp turmeric powder

½ tsp grated fresh ginger

2 tbsp water (to thin the dressing)

¼ tsp sea salt

1. Preheat the oven to 400°F (200°C). Toss sweet potatoes, beets, carrots, and parsnips with olive oil and sea salt. Spread on a baking sheet and roast for 25-30 minutes, flipping halfway.

2. In a small bowl, whisk together tahini, olive oil, lemon juice, turmeric, ginger, sea salt, and water until smooth. Adjust consistency with more water if needed.

3. Lightly sauté or steam cauliflower rice for 2-3 minutes until tender.

4. Divide cauliflower rice into bowls, top with roasted root vegetables, and sprinkle with pumpkin and sunflower seeds.

5. Pour turmeric-tahini dressing over the bowl and serve warm.

Sue Slaughter

Prep Time: 10 minutes

Cook Time: 10-12 minutes

Servings: 2

Ingredients:

2 cups cauliflower rice

1 cup wild mushrooms (shiitake, oyster, maitake), sliced

1 tbsp olive oil or coconut oil

2 cloves garlic, minced

½ cup coconut cream

1 tbsp nutritional yeast (for umami flavor)

1 tsp fresh thyme, chopped

1 tsp fresh sage, chopped

½ tsp sea salt

¼ tsp black pepper (omit for AIP)

Wild Mushroom Risotto with Cauliflower Rice

1. Heat oil in a pan over medium heat. Add mushrooms and cook for 5-7 minutes until softened and golden. Remove and set aside.

2. In the same pan, add minced garlic and sauté for 1 minute. Stir in the cauliflower rice and cook for 3-4 minutes.

3. Pour in the coconut cream, nutritional yeast, thyme, sage, salt, and pepper. Stir well and let simmer for 3-5 minutes until creamy.

4. Fold the sautéed mushrooms back into the risotto, mix well, and serve warm.

Prep Time: 10 minutes

Cook Time: 30 minutes

Servings: 4

Ingredients:

2 acorn squashes, halved and seeds removed

1 cup cooked wild rice

1 tbsp olive oil

½ cup wild mushrooms, chopped (shiitake, cremini, or oyster)

1 cup kale, chopped

¼ cup toasted walnuts, chopped

1 tsp fresh rosemary, minced

1 tsp fresh thyme, minced

½ tsp sea salt

¼ tsp black pepper (omit for AIP)

1 tbsp maple syrup

Stuffed Acorn Squash with Wild Rice & Mushrooms

1. Preheat the oven to 400°F (200°C). Brush squash halves with ½ tbsp olive oil and sprinkle with a pinch of salt. Place cut-side down on a baking sheet and roast for 25-30 minutes, until tender.

2. While the squash is roasting, heat ½ tbsp olive oil in a pan over medium heat. Add mushrooms and sauté for 3-4 minutes until softened. Add kale, rosemary, thyme, salt, and pepper. Sauté for another 2 minutes until kale is wilted.

3. Stir in the cooked wild rice and toasted walnuts, mixing well. Remove from heat.

4. Flip the roasted acorn squash halves over and fill each cavity with the wild rice mixture. Drizzle with maple syrup (if using).

5. For a deeper flavor, return the stuffed squash to the oven for 5 more minutes at 375°F (190°C).

Zucchini Noodle Stir-Fry

Prep Time: 10 minutes

Cook Time: 7-8 minutes

Servings: 2

Ingredients:

2 medium zucchinis, spiralized

1 cup bok choy, chopped

½ cup carrots, julienned

½ cup broccoli florets

½ cup mushrooms, sliced

2 tbsp hemp seeds

For the Sauce

2 tbsp coconut aminos

1 tsp fresh ginger, grated

1 clove garlic, minced

1 tsp raw honey

1. In a small bowl, whisk together coconut aminos, ginger, garlic, and honey. Set aside.

2. Heat a pan over medium heat with a small amount of oil (coconut or olive oil). Add carrots, broccoli, and mushrooms, cooking for 3-4 minutes.

3. Stir in the bok choy and sauce. Cook for another 2 minutes until tender.

4. Add the spiralized zucchini and hemp seeds. Stir-fry for 1-2 minutes until just softened (avoid overcooking).

5. Divide into bowls

Prep Time: 10 minutes

Cook Time: 45 minutes

Servings: 4

Ingredients

1 medium zucchini, thinly sliced

1 medium yellow squash, thinly sliced

1 medium sweet potato, thinly sliced

2 tbsp olive oil

1 tsp fresh thyme, chopped

1 tsp fresh rosemary, chopped

¼ tsp sea salt

¼ cup toasted pine nuts

Roasted Vegetable Tian with Pine Nuts

1. Set to 375°F (190°C).

2. Thinly slice zucchini, yellow squash, and sweet potato into even rounds.

3. In a baking dish, layer the vegetables in an alternating pattern. Drizzle with olive oil, sprinkle with fresh herbs and sea salt.

4. Cover with foil and bake for 30 minutes. Remove foil and bake for an additional 15 minutes, until the edges are golden and tender.

5. Sprinkle toasted pine nuts over the dish before serving.

Sue Slaughter

Prep Time: 10 minutes

Cook Time: 15-18 minutes

Servings: 2

Ingredients:

4 large portobello mushroom caps, stems removed

2 cups fresh spinach, chopped

½ small onion, finely chopped

2 cloves garlic, minced

1 tbsp fresh herbs (parsley, thyme, or basil), chopped

2 tbsp olive oil, divided

¼ cup nutritional yeast

¼ cup toasted walnuts, chopped

½ tsp sea salt

¼ tsp black pepper (omit for AIP)

Stuffed Portobello Mushrooms

1. Set to 375°F (190°C).

2. Wipe clean and remove stems. Place caps on a baking sheet, gill-side up. Drizzle with 1 tbsp olive oil.

3. In a pan, heat 1 tbsp olive oil over medium heat. Add onions and cook for 2-3 minutes until translucent. Stir in garlic, spinach, herbs, salt, and pepper. Sauté for another 2 minutes until spinach is wilted.

4. Spoon the sautéed spinach mixture evenly into the mushroom caps.

5. Sprinkle with nutritional yeast and toasted walnuts. Bake for 15-18 minutes until mushrooms are tender.

6. Drizzle with extra olive oil if desired

Prep Time: 15 minutes

Cook Time: 40 minutes

Servings: 4

Ingredients:

For the Spaghetti Squash

1 medium spaghetti squash

1 tbsp olive oil

½ tsp sea salt

For the Basil-Avocado Pesto

1 cup fresh basil leaves

½ ripe avocado

¼ cup olive oil

1 tbsp lemon juice

2 tbsp pine nuts

½ tsp sea salt

For the Sautéed Vegetables

1 tbsp olive oil

2 cups kale, chopped

1 cup mushrooms, sliced

For Garnish

2 tbsp toasted pumpkin seeds

Spaghetti Squash with Basil-Avocado Pesto

1. Roast the Spaghetti Squash

Preheat the oven to 400°F (200°C).

Cut the spaghetti squash in half lengthwise and remove seeds.

Drizzle with olive oil and sprinkle with sea salt.

Place cut-side down on a baking sheet and roast for 35-40 minutes, or until tender.

Once cooled, use a fork to scrape the flesh into spaghetti-like strands.

2. In a food processor, blend basil, avocado, olive oil, lemon juice, pine nuts, and sea salt until smooth.

3. Sauté the Vegetables

Heat olive oil in a pan over medium heat.

Add mushrooms and cook for 3-4 minutes until softened.

Add kale and cook for another 2 minutes until wilted.

4. Assemble the Dish

Toss the spaghetti squash with the pesto sauce.

Mix in the sautéed kale and mushrooms.

Sprinkle toasted pumpkin seeds on top before serving.

Sue Slaughter

Prep Time: 10 minutes

Cook Time: 15 minutes

Servings: 4

Ingredients:

Base:

1 can (14 oz) full-fat coconut milk

3 cups vegetable or bone broth

1 tbsp coconut oil

1-inch fresh ginger, grated

2 cloves garlic, minced

1 tsp turmeric powder

1 tsp sea salt

Vegetables:**

1 medium carrot, diced

1 small sweet potato, diced

1 cup cauliflower florets

2 cups fresh spinach

To Serve:

2 cups cauliflower rice, steamed

Fresh cilantro, chopped

1 lime, cut into wedges

Coconut Curry Vegetable Soup

1. In a large pot, heat coconut oil over medium heat. Add garlic, ginger, and turmeric. Sauté for 1 minute until fragrant.

2. Add carrots, sweet potatoes, and cauliflower. Stir to coat with spices. Pour in the broth and bring to a gentle simmer. Cook for 10-12 minutes until the vegetables are tender.

3. Stir in coconut milk and spinach. Simmer for another 2-3 minutes until the spinach is wilted.

4. Divide steamed cauliflower rice into bowls, ladle the soup over it, and garnish with fresh cilantro and a squeeze of lime.

Prep Time: 10 minutes

Cook Time: 40-45 minutes

Servings: 2

Ingredients:

2 medium sweet potatoes

2 cups fresh spinach, chopped

¼ cup olives, sliced (Kalamata or green)

1 tbsp capers, rinsed

1 tbsp fresh herbs (parsley, oregano), chopped

1 tbsp olive oil

Tahini Drizzle**

2 tbsp tahini

1 tbsp lemon juice

1 tbsp water

¼ tsp sea salt

¼ tsp garlic powder (omit for AIP)

Mediterranean Stuffed Sweet Potatoes

1. Preheat the oven to 400°F (200°C). Pierce sweet potatoes with a fork and bake for 40-45 minutes until tender.

2. While the potatoes bake, heat olive oil in a pan over medium heat. Sauté spinach for 1-2 minutes until wilted, then add olives, capers, and herbs. Stir for another minute, then remove from heat.

3. In a small bowl, whisk together tahini, lemon juice, water, sea salt, and garlic powder until smooth.

4. Slice sweet potatoes open and fluff the flesh with a fork. Spoon the spinach mixture into each potato and drizzle with tahini sauce. Garnish with fresh parsley.

Sue Slaughter

Prep Time: 10 minutes.

Cook Time: 45 minutes

Servings: 4

Ingredients:

2 cups butternut squash, peeled and cubed

1 cup wild rice, rinsed

¼ cup toasted pecans, chopped

¼ cup dried cranberries (unsweetened)

1 tbsp fresh sage, chopped

1 tbsp fresh thyme leaves

2 tbsp olive oil (divided)

1 tbsp apple cider vinegar

½ tsp sea salt

Butternut Squash and Wild Rice Pilaf

1. Preheat the oven to 400°F (200°C). Toss squash cubes with 1 tbsp olive oil and a pinch of sea salt. Spread on a baking sheet and roast for 20-25 minutes until tender and lightly caramelized.

2. In a pot, bring 2 ½ cups of water to a boil. Add wild rice and a pinch of salt. Reduce heat, cover, and simmer for 40-45 minutes until rice is tender. Drain any excess water.

3. In a small bowl, whisk together apple cider vinegar, remaining olive oil, and a pinch of salt.

4. In a large bowl, combine cooked wild rice, roasted butternut squash, toasted pecans, dried cranberries, and fresh herbs. Drizzle with the dressing and toss to combine.

Prep Time: 10 minutes

Cook Time: 30-35 minutes

Servings: 2-3

Ingredients:

1 large head of cauliflower (cut into thick steaks)

2 tbsp olive oil

2 cups fresh herbs (parsley, cilantro, or basil)

2 tbsp olive oil

Juice of 1 lemon

2 medium sweet potatoes, peeled and chopped

1 tbsp olive oil (for mashed sweet potatoes)

¼ cup coconut milk

2 tbsp toasted pine nuts

Sea salt and black pepper (omit for AIP)

Cauliflower Steaks with Herb Sauce

1. Preheat the oven to 400°F (200°C).

2. Slice the cauliflower into 1-inch thick steaks, ensuring they stay intact. Brush both sides with olive oil and season with a pinch of sea salt.

3. Place the cauliflower steaks on a baking sheet and roast for 20-25 minutes, flipping halfway through, until golden brown and tender.

4. While the cauliflower roasts, blend the fresh herbs, olive oil, and lemon juice in a food processor until smooth. Adjust seasoning to taste with sea salt and pepper.

5. In a medium pot, boil the sweet potatoes until fork-tender, about 15-20 minutes. Drain and return to the pot. Mash with olive oil, coconut milk, and a pinch of sea salt until smooth.

6. Plate the cauliflower steaks, drizzle with herb sauce, and garnish with toasted pine nuts. Serve alongside the mashed sweet potatoes.

Sue Slaughter

Prep Time: 10 minutes

Servings: 2

Ingredients:

Base:

4 cups mixed greens (e.g., spinach, arugula, or lettuce)

Toppings:

1 cucumber, thinly sliced

1 carrot, julienned

1 avocado, sliced

1 small mango, diced

Protein:

¼ cup toasted cashews (or sunflower seeds for AIP)

Sauce:

2 tbsp coconut aminos

Juice of 1 lime

1-inch piece fresh ginger, grated

1 tsp honey

Summer Roll Bowls

1. Arrange mixed greens in a large bowl as the base.

2. Layer sliced cucumber, julienned carrot, avocado, and diced mango on top of the greens.

3. In a small skillet, lightly toast the cashews over low heat for 2-3 minutes, stirring occasionally to avoid burning.

4. In a small bowl, whisk together coconut aminos, lime juice, grated ginger, and honey (if using).

5. Sprinkle the toasted cashews over the bowl and drizzle with the ginger-lime sauce.

6. Toss lightly or enjoy as is, with the sauce on top.

Warm Quinoa and Roasted Vegetable Bowl

Prep Time: 10 minutes

Cook Time: 30 minutes

Servings: 2

Ingredients:

1 cup cooked quinoa (if tolerated)

2 medium carrots, peeled and diced

2 medium beets, peeled and diced

1 medium sweet potato, peeled and diced

2 cups kale, chopped

2 tbsp olive oil

1 tbsp coconut oil

2 tbsp pumpkin seeds, toasted

2 tbsp tahini

1 tsp ground turmeric

1 tbsp lemon juice

1 tbsp water

Sea salt and black pepper (omit pepper for AIP)

1. Preheat the oven to 400°F (200°C). Toss carrots, beets, and sweet potatoes in 1 tbsp olive oil, season with sea salt, and place on a baking sheet. Roast for 20-25 minutes, or until tender and slightly caramelized.

2. While the vegetables roast, heat coconut oil in a skillet over medium heat. Add chopped kale and sauté for 3-5 minutes until wilted. Season with a pinch of sea salt.

3. In a small bowl, whisk together tahini, turmeric, lemon juice, water, and a pinch of salt to form a smooth dressing.

4. In each bowl, layer cooked quinoa, roasted vegetables, sautéed kale, and drizzle with turmeric-tahini dressing.

5. Sprinkle toasted pumpkin seeds on top for added crunch and nutrition.

Sue Slaughter

Spaghetti Squash Pad Thai

Prep Time: 10 minutes

Cook Time: 40 minutes

Servings: 2-3

Ingredients:

1 medium spaghetti squash

1 large carrot, julienned

1 cup broccoli florets

2 scallions, chopped

¼ cup toasted cashews, roughly chopped

For the sauce**:

2 tbsp coconut aminos

1 tbsp lime juice

1 tsp honey (optional, or use a pinch of stevia for AIP)

1 tsp fresh ginger, grated

1. Preheat the oven to 400°F (200°C). Slice the spaghetti squash in half lengthwise and scoop out the seeds. Place the halves cut-side down on a baking sheet lined with parchment paper. Roast for 35-40 minutes until tender. Once cooled, use a fork to shred the flesh into spaghetti-like strands.

2. While the squash is roasting, julienne the carrot, chop the broccoli into small florets, and slice the scallions.

3. Heat a small pan over medium heat and toast the cashews for 2-3 minutes until fragrant and lightly browned.

4. In a small bowl, whisk together coconut aminos, lime juice, honey, and grated ginger until well combined.

5. In a large bowl, toss the roasted spaghetti squash, carrots, broccoli, and scallions. Drizzle with the prepared sauce and toss until evenly coated.

6. Top with toasted cashews and serve

Prep Time: 15 minutes

Cook Time: 25 minutes (for roasting sweet potatoes and cooking rice)

Servings: 2-3 wraps per person

Ingredients:

6 large collard green leaves, blanched (see instructions)

1 cup cooked wild rice

1 small roasted sweet potato, cubed

1 avocado, sliced

¼ cup fresh cilantro, chopped

¼ cup fresh mint, chopped

2 tbsp tahini

1 tbsp lemon juice

1 tsp water

½ tsp sea salt

Stuffed Collard Green Wraps

1. To blanch the collard green leaves, bring a large pot of water to a boil. Trim the tough stems from the leaves and blanch them for 30 seconds to 1 minute. Remove and transfer to an ice bath to stop the cooking process. Pat dry with a paper towel.

2. In a bowl, combine the cooked wild rice, roasted sweet potato cubes, avocado slices, cilantro, and mint. Mix gently to combine.

3. In a small bowl, whisk together tahini, lemon juice, water (if needed), and sea salt. Adjust the consistency with more water if the sauce is too thick.

4. Place a blanched collard green leaf flat on a surface. Add a spoonful of the wild rice and sweet potato filling in the center, then fold the sides of the leaf over the filling and roll it up tightly, like a burrito. Repeat for the remaining leaves.

5. Serve the wraps with a side of tahini-lemon dipping sauce.

Sue Slaughter

Prep Time: 15 minutes

Cook Time: 40-45 minutes

Servings: 4

Ingredients:

2 large carrots, peeled and cut into sticks

2 parsnips, peeled and cut into sticks

2 medium sweet potatoes, peeled and cut into cubes

2 medium beets, peeled and cut into cubes

2 tbsp maple syrup

2 tbsp olive oil

1 tsp ground cinnamon

1 tsp ground ginger

½ cup toasted walnuts, chopped

1 tbsp fresh thyme, chopped

4 cups cauliflower florets

1 tbsp olive oil

Sea salt and pepper, to taste

Maple-Glazed Root Vegetables with Cauliflower Mash

1. Preheat the oven to 400°F (200°C). Place carrots, parsnips, sweet potatoes, and beets on a baking sheet.

2. In a small bowl, whisk together maple syrup, olive oil, cinnamon, and ginger. Drizzle the glaze over the root vegetables and toss to coat evenly.

3. Roast in the preheated oven for 30-35 minutes, flipping halfway through, until vegetables are tender and caramelized.

4. While the vegetables roast, steam cauliflower florets for 10-12 minutes, or until tender. Mash the cauliflower with olive oil, salt, and pepper until smooth.

5. Once the root vegetables are roasted, plate them over the cauliflower mash. Top with toasted walnuts and fresh thyme.

Prep Time: 10 minutes

Cook Time: 5 minutes (for steaming broccoli)

Servings: 2

Ingredients:

2 medium zucchinis, spiralized

For the sauce:

1 ripe avocado

2 tbsp fresh basil, chopped

2 tbsp olive oil

1 tbsp lemon juice

¼ tsp sea salt

¼ tsp black pepper (omit for AIP)

1 cup broccoli florets, steamed

2 tbsp toasted pine nuts

Fresh herbs (parsley or basil)

Zucchini Pasta with Avocado Cream Sauce

1. Use a spiralizer to turn the zucchinis into noodles. If you don't have a spiralizer, you can use a vegetable peeler to create thin strips.

2. In a blender or food processor, combine avocado, basil, olive oil, lemon juice, salt, and pepper. Blend until smooth and creamy.

3. In a steamer basket, steam the broccoli florets for 4-5 minutes, or until tender but still vibrant green.

4. Toss the zucchini noodles with the avocado cream sauce until well coated.

5. Plate the zucchini pasta, top with steamed broccoli, toasted pine nuts, and garnish with fresh herbs.

Prep Time: 10 minutes

Cook Time: 15-20 minutes

Servings: 4

Ingredients:

4 cups cauliflower rice (fresh or frozen)

2 tbsp olive oil

1 cup wild mushrooms, sliced (e.g., shiitake, cremini, or chanterelle)

1 bunch asparagus, trimmed and cut into 1-inch pieces

½ cup coconut cream

2 cloves garlic, minced

1 tbsp fresh thyme, chopped

1 tbsp fresh parsley, chopped

2 tbsp nutritional yeast

½ tsp sea salt

¼ tsp black pepper (omit for AIP)

Wild Mushroom and Asparagus Risotto

1. If using fresh cauliflower, pulse it in a food processor until it resembles rice. Set aside.

2. Heat olive oil in a large pan over medium heat. Add garlic and sauté for 1 minute. Stir in the mushrooms and asparagus, and cook until softened, about 5-7 minutes.

3. Add the cauliflower rice to the pan with the mushrooms and asparagus. Stir well to combine and cook for about 5 minutes, until the cauliflower rice is tender.

4. Pour in the coconut cream, nutritional yeast, thyme, parsley, salt, and pepper. Stir and cook for another 2-3 minutes, allowing the cream to incorporate into the rice.

5. Plate the risotto, garnish with additional herbs if desired, and serve warm.

Warm Brussels Sprout and Apple Salad

Prep Time: 10 minutes

Cook Time: 10 minutes

Servings: 2-4

Ingredients:

4 cups shaved Brussels sprouts (about 1 lb)

1 apple, diced (preferably a sweet variety like Fuji or Honeycrisp)

¼ cup toasted walnuts, roughly chopped

2 tbsp apple cider vinegar

1 tbsp maple syrup

2 tbsp olive oil

Salt and pepper to taste (omit pepper for AIP)

2 cups cooked quinoa or cauliflower rice

1. In a dry skillet, toast the walnuts over medium heat for about 3-5 minutes until fragrant and slightly browned. Remove from heat and set aside.

2. Heat 1 tbsp olive oil in a large pan over medium heat. Add the shaved Brussels sprouts and sauté for 5-7 minutes until softened and lightly browned. Stir occasionally to avoid burning.

3. In a small bowl, whisk together the apple cider vinegar, maple syrup, and remaining olive oil. Season with salt and pepper (if using).

4. Once the Brussels sprouts are sautéed, add the diced apples to the pan and cook for 1-2 minutes until slightly softened.

5. Remove from heat and toss the Brussels sprouts and apple mixture with the dressing. Top with toasted walnuts.

6. Serve the salad warm over a bed of quinoa or cauliflower rice, if desired.

Sue Slaughter

SEAFOODS

Herb-Roasted Wild Salmon with Lemon

Prep Time: 10 minutes

Cook Time: 15 minutes

Servings: 4

Ingredients:

4 wild-caught salmon fillets (about 6 oz each)

2 tbsp fresh dill, chopped

2 tbsp fresh parsley, chopped

2 tbsp fresh thyme, chopped

1 lemon, thinly sliced

2 tbsp olive oil

2 cloves garlic, minced

Sea salt and black pepper (omit black pepper for AIP)

1. Preheat your oven to 375°F (190°C).

2. Place the salmon fillets on a baking sheet lined with parchment paper. Drizzle olive oil over the fillets and rub gently to coat.

3. Sprinkle fresh dill, parsley, thyme, minced garlic (if using), and sea salt over the salmon. Place lemon slices on top of the fillets.

4. Roast the salmon in the preheated oven for 12-15 minutes, or until the salmon is cooked through and flakes easily with a fork.

5. Plate the salmon and serve with steamed asparagus and cauliflower rice on the side.

Sue Slaughter

Prep Time: 10 minutes

Cook Time: 15-18 minutes

Servings: 4

Ingredients:

4 wild-caught cod fillets (about 4 oz each)

1-inch piece fresh ginger, sliced

2 cloves garlic, smashed

2 tbsp coconut aminos

2 heads bok choy, chopped

2 green onions, sliced

2 cups bone broth (chicken or vegetable)

1 tbsp olive oil

Fresh cilantro, chopped

Ginger-Poached Cod with Bok Choy

1. In a large skillet or shallow pan, combine bone broth, ginger, garlic, and coconut aminos. Bring to a simmer over medium heat.

2. Add the cod fillets to the poaching liquid, making sure the fish is mostly submerged. Cover and let simmer for 10-12 minutes, or until the fish is fully cooked and flakes easily with a fork.

3. While the cod is poaching, heat a separate pan with a small amount of olive oil over medium heat. Add the bok choy and green onions, sautéing for 3-4 minutes until the bok choy is tender but still crisp.

4. Once the cod is cooked, carefully remove it from the pan and place it on serving plates. Drizzle with a little olive oil and top with sautéed bok choy and green onions. Garnish with fresh cilantro.

Prep Time: 10 minutes

Cook Time: 15 minutes

Servings: 4

Ingredients:

4 wild-caught sole fillets

½ cup almond flour (for coating)

2 tbsp fresh parsley, chopped

1 tbsp fresh thyme, chopped

1 tbsp fresh oregano, chopped

Zest of 1 lemon

2 tbsp olive oil (divided)

Sea salt and black pepper to taste (omit black pepper for AIP)

2 medium zucchinis, spiralized into noodles or sliced into thin strips

Baked Sole with Herb Crust and Sautéed Zucchini Noodles

1. In a shallow dish, combine almond flour, chopped parsley, thyme, oregano, lemon zest, salt, and pepper.

2. Brush both sides of each sole fillet with 1 tbsp olive oil. Dredge the fillets in the almond flour mixture, pressing gently to ensure the herbs stick to the fish.

3. Preheat the oven to 375°F (190°C). Place the coated sole fillets on a baking sheet lined with parchment paper. Drizzle with a little olive oil and bake for 10-12 minutes, or until the fish flakes easily with a fork.

4. While the fish is baking, heat the remaining 1 tbsp olive oil in a pan over medium heat. Add the zucchini noodles and sauté for 2-3 minutes, just until slightly tender. Season with salt to taste.

5. Plate the baked sole fillets with the sautéed zucchini noodles on the side.

Sue Slaughter

Prep Time: 10 minutes

Cook Time: 15 minutes

Servings: 4

Ingredients:

4 black cod fillets (about 4-6 oz each)

2 tbsp white miso paste (if tolerated; substitute with coconut aminos for AIP)

1 tbsp honey or maple syrup

2 tbsp coconut aminos

1-inch piece fresh ginger, grated

1 tbsp olive oil

1 cup steamed broccoli

1 cup steamed carrots

Miso-Glazed Black Cod

1. In a small bowl, whisk together the white miso paste, honey (or maple syrup), coconut aminos, and grated ginger until smooth.

2. Pat the black cod fillets dry with paper towels. Brush both sides of the fillets with the miso glaze and set aside to marinate for 10 minutes (if time allows).

3. Heat olive oil in a skillet over medium-high heat. Once hot, add the cod fillets and cook for about 3-4 minutes per side, until the fish is golden brown and cooked through.

4. While the fish is cooking, steam the broccoli and carrots until tender (about 5-7 minutes).

5. Plate the black cod fillets with the steamed broccoli and carrots. Drizzle any remaining glaze over the fish.

Prep Time: 10 minutes

Cook Time: 6-8 minutes

Servings: 2

Ingredients:

4 fresh sardines, cleaned and gutted

2 tbsp olive oil

1 lemon, sliced

1 cup shaved fennel

1 small celery stalk, thinly sliced

1 small carrot, grated or julienned

2 tbsp fresh parsley, chopped

2 tbsp fresh dill, chopped

2 tbsp apple cider vinegar

1 tbsp olive oil

½ tsp sea salt

¼ tsp black pepper (omit for AIP)

Grilled Sardines with Fennel Slaw

1. In a bowl, combine shaved fennel, celery, carrot, parsley, and dill. In a small jar, mix apple cider vinegar, olive oil, salt, and pepper. Shake or whisk to combine, then pour over the slaw and toss to coat. Set aside.

2. Preheat the grill or grill pan over medium heat. Brush the sardines with olive oil and season with a pinch of sea salt and black pepper.

3. Place the sardines on the grill and cook for 2-3 minutes per side, or until they are golden and crispy on the outside.

4. Plate the grilled sardines, squeeze lemon juice over the top, and serve with the fennel slaw on the side.

Coconut-Poached Halibut

Prep Time: 10 minutes

Cook Time: 15-20 minutes

Servings: 4

Ingredients:

4 wild-caught halibut fillets (about 6 oz each)

1 can (13.5 oz) full-fat coconut milk

1 stalk lemongrass, bruised and chopped into large pieces

1-inch piece fresh ginger, sliced

3-4 lime leaves (optional)

1 tbsp olive oil

1 cup cauliflower rice

2 cups sautéed greens like spinach, kale, or Swiss chard

½ tsp sea salt

1 tbsp fresh cilantro, chopped

1. In a large, shallow pan, combine coconut milk, lemongrass, ginger, lime leaves, and sea salt. Bring to a gentle simmer over medium heat.

2. Add the halibut fillets to the pan, ensuring they're partially submerged in the coconut milk. Cover and simmer for 10-12 minutes, or until the fish is cooked through and flakes easily with a fork.

3. While the fish is poaching, heat olive oil in a separate pan over medium heat. Add cauliflower rice and sauté for 5-7 minutes until tender. Season with a pinch of salt if desired.

4. In the same pan, sauté the greens for 3-4 minutes until wilted.

5. Plate the halibut fillets with a side of cauliflower rice and sautéed greens. Spoon some of the coconut broth over the fish and garnish with fresh cilantro.

Herbed Scallops with Roasted Root Vegetables

Prep Time: 10 minutes

Cook Time: 30-35 minutes

Servings: 3-4

Ingredients:

12-16 sea scallops (fresh or thawed)

2 tbsp fresh thyme, chopped

2 tbsp fresh rosemary, chopped

2 tbsp olive oil (divided)

1 tbsp garlic-infused oil

3 carrots, peeled and cut into chunks

2 parsnips, peeled and cut into chunks

1 large sweet potato, peeled and cut into chunks

Sea salt, to taste

Fresh ground black pepper (omit for AIP)

1. Preheat the oven to 400°F (200°C). In a large bowl, toss the carrots, parsnips, and sweet potato chunks with 1 tablespoon of olive oil and a pinch of sea salt. Spread them evenly on a baking sheet.

2. Roast the vegetables in the preheated oven for 25-30 minutes, flipping halfway through, until they are tender and slightly caramelized.

3. While the vegetables are roasting, pat the scallops dry with a paper towel and season with a pinch of sea salt and freshly ground black pepper (if using).

4. Heat 1 tablespoon of olive oil in a large skillet over medium-high heat. Add the scallops to the pan and cook for 2-3 minutes per side until golden brown and just cooked through (opaque in the center).

5. Once the scallops are cooked, drizzle them with garlic-infused oil and sprinkle with fresh thyme and rosemary. Serve with roasted root vegetables on the side.

Sue Slaughter

Baked Mackerel with Herbs

Prep Time: 10 minutes

Cook Time: 15-20 minutes

Servings: 2

Ingredients:

2 fresh mackerel fillets

1 tbsp fresh dill, chopped

1 tbsp fresh parsley, chopped

1 lemon, sliced

2 tbsp olive oil

2 cloves garlic, minced

Sea salt and black pepper to taste (omit for AIP)

1. Preheat your oven to 375°F (190°C).

2. Place the mackerel fillets on a baking sheet lined with parchment paper. Drizzle with olive oil and season with sea salt and black pepper (if using).

3. Sprinkle fresh dill and parsley over the mackerel. If using, add minced garlic on top of the fillets.

4. Place lemon slices on and around the fillets.

5. Bake in the preheated oven for 15-20 minutes, or until the fish is cooked through and flakes easily with a fork.

6. Serve the baked mackerel with a side of steamed vegetables and a green salad for a complete meal.

Prep Time: 10 minutes

Cook Time: 10-12 minutes

Servings: 2

Ingredients:

2 fresh tuna steaks (about 6 oz each)

1-inch piece fresh ginger, grated

3 scallions, thinly sliced

2 tbsp coconut aminos

1 tbsp olive oil

1 tsp sesame oil (optional, if tolerated)

2 cups bok choy, chopped

1 tbsp olive oil

1 ½ cups cauliflower rice (fresh or frozen)

½ tsp sea salt

¼ tsp black pepper (omit for AIP)

Tuna Steak with Ginger-Scallion Sauce

1. In a small bowl, combine grated ginger, sliced scallions, coconut aminos, and sesame oil (if using). Set aside.

2. Heat olive oil in a pan over medium-high heat. Season the tuna steaks with salt and pepper (omit pepper for AIP). Sear the tuna steaks for 2-3 minutes per side for rare, or longer if desired. Remove from heat and set aside.

3. In a separate pan, heat 1 tbsp olive oil over medium heat. Add chopped bok choy and sauté for 3-4 minutes, until tender. Season with a pinch of salt.

4. In a pan over medium heat, sauté cauliflower rice for 3-4 minutes until tender, adding salt to taste.

5. Plate the tuna steaks and drizzle with the ginger-scallion sauce. Serve with sautéed bok choy and cauliflower rice on the side.

Sue Slaughter

Prep Time: 10 minutes

Cook Time: 20 minutes

Servings: 4

Seafood and Sweet Potato Stew

Ingredients:

1 lb mixed seafood (shrimp, white fish, scallops)

1 medium sweet potato, peeled and diced

1 small onion, chopped

1 carrot, diced

1 celery stalk, diced

1-inch piece fresh ginger, grated

1-inch piece fresh turmeric, grated or ½ tsp ground turmeric

2 cups bone broth

1 cup coconut milk (full-fat, canned)

1 tbsp olive oil or coconut oil

1 tsp sea salt

½ tsp black pepper (omit for AIP)

2 tbsp fresh herbs (parsley, cilantro, or basil), chopped

1. Heat oil in a large pot over medium heat. Add onion, carrot, and celery. Sauté for 3-4 minutes until softened.

2. Stir in grated ginger and turmeric. Cook for 1 minute until fragrant.

3. Pour in the bone broth and bring to a gentle simmer. Add the diced sweet potatoes and cook for 10 minutes until tender.

4. Add the mixed seafood to the pot and cook for another 5-7 minutes until the shrimp is pink and the fish flakes easily.

5. Stir in the coconut milk, sea salt, and black pepper. Simmer for 2 more minutes, then remove from heat.

6. Stir in fresh herbs and serve warm.

Wild Salmon and Fennel Soup

Prep Time: 10 minutes

Cook Time: 15-20 minutes

Servings: 4

Ingredients:

2 cups bone broth (chicken or fish)

1 can (13.5 oz) coconut milk

1 fennel bulb, thinly sliced

1 small onion, diced

1 celery stalk, diced

8 oz wild salmon, cut into bite-sized pieces

2 tbsp fresh dill, chopped

1 tbsp olive oil

½ tsp sea salt

¼ tsp black pepper (omit for AIP)

Juice of ½ lemon

1. In a large pot, heat olive oil over medium heat. Add onion, fennel, and celery. Sauté for 3-4 minutes until softened.

2. Pour in bone broth and bring to a gentle simmer. Let cook for 10 minutes.

3. Stir in coconut milk and bring to a low simmer. Add salmon pieces and let cook for 5-7 minutes, until salmon is opaque and flakes easily.

4. Stir in dill, lemon juice, salt, and pepper. Remove from heat.

5. Ladle into bowls

Sue Slaughter

Prep Time: 10 minutes

Cook Time: 20 minutes

Servings: 4

Ingredients:

1 lb mixed seafood (shrimp, white fish, mussels, clams, etc.), cleaned and prepped

1 medium onion, diced

2 celery stalks, diced

2 carrots, peeled and diced

1 bulb fennel, thinly sliced

4 cups fish stock or bone broth

2 tbsp fresh basil, chopped

2 tbsp fresh oregano, chopped

2 tbsp fresh parsley, chopped

Pinch of saffron (optional)

2 tbsp olive oil

Sea salt and black pepper (omit black pepper for AIP)

Cioppino-Inspired Seafood Soup (Nightshade-Free)

1. Heat olive oil in a large pot over medium heat. Add diced onion, celery, carrots, and fennel. Sauté for 5-7 minutes until softened.

2. Pour in the fish stock or bone broth and bring to a simmer. Stir in the fresh basil, oregano, parsley, and saffron (if using). Season with sea salt and black pepper (if using). Let the broth simmer for about 10 minutes to meld the flavors.

3. Add the mixed seafood to the pot and cook for an additional 5-7 minutes, or until the shrimp turns pink and the mussels and clams open up.

4. Ladle the soup into bowls and garnish with additional fresh herbs if desired.

Shrimp and Avocado Lettuce Cups

Prep Time: 10 minutes

Servings: 2-3

Ingredients:

12 oz wild-caught shrimp, cooked and peeled

1 ripe avocado, diced

½ cucumber, diced

1 small carrot, julienned

2 tbsp fresh cilantro, chopped

2 tbsp fresh mint, chopped

8-10 butter lettuce leaves

For the dressing:

1 tbsp lime juice

2 tbsp olive oil

1 tsp fresh grated ginger

1 tsp honey (optional, or use a pinch of stevia for a low-sugar option)

1. In a large bowl, combine the cooked shrimp, diced avocado, cucumber, carrot, cilantro, and mint. Toss gently to combine.

2. In a small bowl, whisk together lime juice, olive oil, grated ginger, and honey (if using).

3. Spoon the shrimp and avocado mixture into the center of each butter lettuce leaf.

4. Drizzle the dressing over the shrimp and avocado mixture.

5. Arrange the filled lettuce cups on a plate and serve

Sue Slaughter

Smoked Salmon Bowl

Prep Time: 10 minutes

Cook Time: 6-8 minutes (for the eggs)

Servings: 1

Ingredients:

3 oz smoked wild salmon

1 cup sautéed greens (kale or spinach)

½ avocado, sliced

2 soft-boiled pasture-raised eggs (optional, depending on tolerance)

1 tbsp fresh herbs (parsley, dill, or chives), chopped

1 tbsp olive oil

1 tbsp lemon juice

Sea salt (to taste)

Freshly cracked black pepper (omit for AIP)

1. Heat a small amount of olive oil in a skillet over medium heat. Add the kale or spinach and sauté for 3-4 minutes, or until wilted. Set aside.

2. If using eggs, bring a small pot of water to a boil. Lower the eggs in and cook for 6-7 minutes for soft-boiled eggs. Drain and set aside. Peel the eggs once cool enough to handle.

3. In a bowl, layer the sautéed greens, smoked salmon, avocado slices, and soft-boiled eggs (if using).

4. In a small bowl, whisk together olive oil, lemon juice, sea salt, and pepper.

5. Drizzle the dressing over the assembled bowl and top with fresh herbs.

Prep Time: 10 minutes

Servings: 2

Sardine and Cucumber Salad

Ingredients:

1 can wild sardines in olive oil (drained)

1 medium cucumber, sliced

½ small red onion, thinly sliced (soaked in water for 10 minutes to reduce intensity)

2 tbsp fresh dill, chopped

1 tbsp lemon juice

2 tbsp olive oil

3 cups mixed greens like arugula, spinach, or lettuce

½ tsp sea salt

¼ tsp black pepper (omit for AIP)

1. Soak the thinly sliced red onion in water for about 10 minutes to mellow its intensity. Drain well.

2. In a large bowl, combine the cucumber, red onion, fresh dill, and sardines (including some of the olive oil from the can).

3. In a small bowl, whisk together lemon juice, olive oil, salt, and black pepper (if using). Pour over the salad and toss gently to combine.

4. Arrange the mixed greens on a plate or in a bowl and top with the sardine mixture.

Prep Time: 10 minutes

Cook Time: (marinating time of 20-30 minutes)

Servings: 2-3

Ingredients:

8 oz wild-caught white fish (like cod, halibut) and/or shrimp, diced

½ cup fresh lime juice (about 3-4 limes)

1 avocado, diced

1 small cucumber, diced

¼ cup red onion, finely chopped

¼ cup fresh cilantro, chopped

1 tbsp olive oil

Sea salt and black pepper (omit pepper for AIP)

Lettuce cups or plantain chips for serving

Seafood and Avocado Ceviche

1. In a medium bowl, combine the diced fish and/or shrimp with fresh lime juice. Stir to coat the seafood, ensuring it's fully covered. Cover and refrigerate for 20-30 minutes until the seafood "cooks" in the lime juice (the fish will become opaque).

2. After the seafood is marinated, add the diced avocado, cucumber, red onion, cilantro, olive oil, and a pinch of sea salt to the bowl. Gently stir to combine, being careful not to mash the avocado.

3. Spoon the ceviche mixture into lettuce cups or serve with plantain chips on the side.

Prep Time: 15 minutes (plus 15-minute marinating time)

Cook Time: 10 minutes

Servings: 2

Ingredients:

1 lb wild-caught shrimp, peeled and deveined

1 cup fresh pineapple chunks

½ red onion, cut into chunks

For the marinade:

3 tbsp coconut aminos

1 tbsp fresh ginger, grated

2 cloves garlic, minced

1 tbsp honey

2 cups cauliflower rice

Olive oil

Fresh cilantro

Grilled Shrimp and Pineapple Skewers

1. In a small bowl, combine coconut aminos, grated ginger, minced garlic, and honey. Mix well.

2. Place the shrimp in a shallow dish and pour the marinade over them. Toss to coat evenly and refrigerate for at least 15 minutes.

3. Thread the marinated shrimp, pineapple chunks, and red onion onto skewers, alternating each ingredient.

4. Preheat the grill or grill pan over medium heat. Lightly brush with olive oil to prevent sticking. Grill the skewers for about 2-3 minutes per side or until the shrimp are cooked through and pink.

5. While grilling, heat a skillet over medium heat with a little olive oil. Add cauliflower rice and cook for 5-7 minutes, stirring occasionally, until soft and slightly browned.

6. Place the grilled skewers on a plate and serve alongside the cauliflower rice. Garnish with fresh cilantro if desired.

Prep Time: 10 minutes

Cook Time: 6 minutes

Servings: 2

Ingredients:

6 large sea scallops, cleaned

2 medium cucumbers, spiralized into noodles

1 small carrot, sliced into ribbons

¼ cup fresh mint, chopped

¼ cup fresh cilantro, chopped

For the dressing:

2 tbsp lime juice (freshly squeezed)

2 tbsp olive oil

1 tsp fresh ginger, grated

1 tsp honey

Scallop and Cucumber Noodle Salad

1. In a large bowl, combine the spiralized cucumber noodles, carrot ribbons, mint, and cilantro. Set aside.

2. In a small bowl, whisk together lime juice, olive oil, ginger, and honey until well combined.

3. Heat a skillet over medium-high heat. Lightly season the scallops with sea salt and black pepper (omit black pepper for AIP). Add 1 tbsp olive oil to the pan, then sear the scallops for 2-3 minutes per side, until golden and opaque.

4. Toss the cucumber and carrot mixture with the dressing. Plate the salad and top with the seared scallops.

5. Garnish with additional fresh mint and cilantro, if desired.

Prep Time: 10 minutes

Cook Time: 10-12 minutes

Servings: 2

Ingredients:

2 ripe avocados, halved and pitted

6 oz wild-caught crab meat (fresh or canned, drained)

½ cucumber, finely diced

¼ red onion, finely diced

2 tbsp fresh cilantro, chopped

2 tbsp fresh parsley, chopped

1 tbsp lime juice

1 tbsp olive oil

Sea salt to taste

Black pepper (omit for AIP)

Baked Stuffed Avocados with Crab

1. In a bowl, combine the crab meat, diced cucumber, red onion, cilantro, parsley, and lime juice. Mix well and season with sea salt.

2. Scoop out a small portion of the avocado flesh to create room for the filling. Stuff each avocado half with the crab mixture.

3. Preheat the oven to 375°F (190°C). Place the stuffed avocado halves on a baking sheet and bake for 10-12 minutes, or until heated through.

4. Drizzle with olive oil before serving and garnish with additional fresh herbs if desired.

Sue Slaughter

POULTRY AND MEAT BASED

Prep Time: 10 minutes (plus marinating time)

Cook Time: 20-25 minutes

Servings: 2

Ingredients:

4 bone-in, skin-on chicken thighs

1 tbsp turmeric powder

1 tbsp fresh ginger, grated (or 1 tbsp ginger paste)

1 tbsp garlic paste

1 cup coconut milk

1 tbsp olive oil or coconut oil

½ tsp sea salt

¼ tsp black pepper (omit for AIP)

2 tbsp fresh cilantro, chopped

2 cups cauliflower rice (fresh or frozen)

Turmeric Ginger Chicken Thighs with Cauliflower Rice

1. In a small bowl, combine turmeric, grated ginger, garlic paste, and coconut milk. Rub the mixture over the chicken thighs, making sure they are evenly coated. Let it marinate for at least 20 minutes, or refrigerate for a few hours for more flavor.

2. Heat olive oil or coconut oil in a large skillet over medium heat. Once hot, add the marinated chicken thighs, skin-side down. Sear for 5-7 minutes until the skin is crispy and golden. Flip the chicken and reduce the heat to low. Cover and cook for another 10-12 minutes, until the chicken is cooked through and the internal temperature reaches 165°F (74°C).

3. While the chicken cooks, heat a separate skillet over medium heat. Add the cauliflower rice and cook for 5-7 minutes, stirring occasionally, until tender. Season with a pinch of salt and pepper.

4. Plate the chicken thighs over the cauliflower rice and garnish with fresh cilantro.

Sue Slaughter

Prep Time: 10 minutes

Cook Time: 10 minutes

Servings: 4

Lemon Herb Turkey Burgers

Ingredients:

1 lb ground pasture-raised turkey

2 tbsp fresh parsley, chopped

2 tbsp fresh mint, chopped

2 tbsp fresh dill, chopped

1 small zucchini, grated (excess water squeezed out)

1 small onion, finely chopped

2 cloves garlic, minced

1 tbsp lemon zest

1 tbsp lemon juice

½ tsp sea salt

¼ tsp black pepper (omit for AIP)

4 large lettuce leaves like romaine or butter lettuce

1 ripe avocado, sliced

1. In a large bowl, combine ground turkey, parsley, mint, dill, grated zucchini, onion, garlic, lemon zest, lemon juice, sea salt, and black pepper. Mix well until all ingredients are evenly incorporated.

2. Divide the mixture into 4 equal portions and shape them into burger patties.

3. Heat a skillet or grill over medium heat. Lightly grease with olive oil or cooking spray. Cook the turkey burgers for 4-5 minutes per side, or until they are fully cooked through (internal temperature should reach 165°F/74°C).

4. Place each turkey patty on a lettuce leaf and top with sliced avocado. Fold the lettuce around the burger to create a wrap.

5. Serve with a side of your choice or enjoy as is.

Prep Time: 10 minutes (plus marinating time)

Cook Time: 35-40 minutes

Servings: 4

Ingredients:

4 chicken breasts or thighs (boneless, skinless)

¼ cup apple cider vinegar

2 tbsp olive oil

3 garlic cloves, minced

2 sprigs fresh thyme or 1 tsp dried thyme

1 tsp sea salt

¼ tsp black pepper (omit for AIP)

2 cups assorted root vegetables like carrots, sweet potatoes, parsnips, chopped

1 tbsp olive oil

Apple Cider Vinegar Chicken with Roasted Root Vegetables

1. In a bowl, combine apple cider vinegar, olive oil, minced garlic, fresh thyme, sea salt, and black pepper (if using). Place the chicken breasts or thighs in the marinade, ensuring they are fully coated. Cover and refrigerate for at least 30 minutes or overnight for maximum flavor.

2. Preheat the oven to 400°F (200°C). Toss the chopped root vegetables with 1 tbsp olive oil and a pinch of salt. Spread them evenly on a baking sheet and roast for 25-30 minutes, or until tender and golden, stirring halfway through.

3. Heat a large skillet over medium heat. Remove the chicken from the marinade (discard any excess marinade) and cook for 5-7 minutes per side, or until fully cooked through and golden brown.

4. Plate the chicken alongside the roasted root vegetables. Garnish with additional fresh thyme if desired.

Sue Slaughter

Prep Time: 10 minutes

Cook Time: 20 minutes

Servings: 2

Coconut Curry Chicken with Cauliflower Rice

Ingredients:

2 boneless, skinless chicken breasts, diced

1 tbsp curry powder (nightshade-free, such as turmeric-based curry powder)

1 cup coconut milk (full-fat)

1 medium onion, chopped

2 cloves garlic, minced

1-inch piece fresh ginger, grated

2 medium carrots, sliced

1 cup broccoli florets

2 tbsp olive oil

1 tsp sea salt

1 tbsp fresh cilantro (optional, for garnish)

2 cups cauliflower rice

1. Heat a non-stick skillet over medium heat. Add the cauliflower rice and cook for 5-7 minutes, stirring occasionally, until tender. Set aside.

2. In a large skillet, heat olive oil over medium heat. Add the chopped onion, garlic, and grated ginger. Sauté for 3-4 minutes, until softened and fragrant.

3. Add the diced chicken breast to the skillet and cook for 5-6 minutes, until browned on all sides.

4. Stir in the carrots and broccoli. Cook for an additional 4-5 minutes, until the vegetables start to soften.

5. Sprinkle the curry powder over the chicken and vegetables. Stir well to coat, then add the coconut milk and sea salt. Bring to a gentle simmer and cook for 10-12 minutes, until the chicken is cooked through and the sauce has thickened.

6. Spoon the curry over a bed of cauliflower rice and garnish with fresh cilantro, if desired.

Prep Time: 10 minutes

Cook Time: 15 minutes

Servings: 2

Ingredients:

2 duck breasts (skin-on)

2 tbsp pure maple syrup

1-inch piece fresh ginger, grated

2 tbsp coconut aminos

2 cups leafy greens (spinach, kale, or Swiss chard), chopped

1 tbsp olive oil

½ tsp sea salt

¼ tsp black pepper (omit for AIP)

Maple-Ginger Glazed Duck Breast with Sautéed Greens

1. In a small bowl, whisk together maple syrup, grated ginger, and coconut aminos until smooth. Set aside.

2. Score the skin of the duck breasts in a crisscross pattern. Heat a large skillet over medium heat. Place the duck breasts skin-side down and cook for 6-7 minutes until the skin is golden and crispy. Flip the breasts and cook for another 4-5 minutes for medium-rare, or longer for your desired doneness. Remove from the pan and set aside to rest.

3. In the same skillet, pour the maple-ginger mixture over the drippings. Bring to a simmer over medium heat and cook for 2-3 minutes, allowing it to thicken slightly.

4. In another pan, heat olive oil over medium heat. Add the chopped leafy greens and sauté for 3-4 minutes until wilted. Season with salt and pepper.

5. Slice the duck breasts and drizzle with the maple-ginger glaze. Serve with the sautéed greens on the side.

Sue Slaughter

Prep Time: 10 minutes

Cook Time: 45-55 minutes

Servings: 2

Ingredients:

2 Cornish game hens (about 1 to 1.5 lbs each)

Zest of 1 orange

Zest of 1 lemon

2 tbsp fresh herbs (rosemary, thyme, or sage), chopped

3 tbsp olive oil

1 medium fennel bulb, sliced

2 medium carrots, peeled and cut into sticks

½ tsp sea salt

¼ tsp black pepper (omit for AIP)

Citrus Herb Cornish Game Hens

1. Preheat your oven to 400°F (200°C).

2. Rinse the Cornish game hens and pat them dry with paper towels. Place them in a roasting pan.

3. In a small bowl, combine orange zest, lemon zest, chopped fresh herbs, olive oil, sea salt, and black pepper. Rub this mixture generously all over the hens.

4. In the same roasting pan, add sliced fennel and carrot sticks around the hens. Drizzle with a bit of olive oil and season with salt and pepper.

5. Roast the hens and vegetables for 45-55 minutes, or until the hens are fully cooked and golden brown. The internal temperature of the hens should reach 165°F (74°C).

6. Remove the hens from the oven and let rest for a few minutes before serving with the roasted fennel and carrots.

Prep Time: 10 minutes (plus marinating time)

Cook Time: 30 minutes

Servings: 4

Ingredients:

4 chicken breasts or thighs, bone-in or boneless

2 tbsp fresh rosemary, chopped

2 tbsp balsamic vinegar

3 cloves garlic, minced

1 tbsp honey

2 tbsp olive oil (divided)

1 lb Brussels sprouts, trimmed and halved

½ tsp sea salt

¼ tsp black pepper (omit for AIP)

Rosemary Balsamic Chicken with Roasted Brussels Sprouts

1. In a small bowl, combine balsamic vinegar, garlic, honey (if using), rosemary, 1 tbsp olive oil, salt, and pepper. Place the chicken in a shallow dish or a ziplock bag, pour the marinade over it, and let it marinate for at least 30 minutes, or up to 4 hours in the fridge.

2. Preheat the oven to 400°F (200°C).

3. Toss the Brussels sprouts with the remaining 1 tbsp olive oil, salt, and pepper. Spread them evenly on a baking sheet.

4. Place the marinated chicken on the baking sheet with the Brussels sprouts, making sure they are spread out in a single layer. Roast for 25-30 minutes, or until the chicken reaches an internal temperature of 165°F (75°C) and the Brussels sprouts are golden and crispy, turning halfway through the cooking time.

5. Plate the rosemary balsamic chicken with the roasted Brussels sprouts. Serve warm.

Sue Slaughter

Prep Time: 10 minutes

Cook Time: 1-1.5 hours

Servings: 4-6

Ingredients:

1 whole chicken (about 3-4 lbs), cleaned and prepared

2-inch piece of fresh ginger, sliced

4 scallions, chopped into large pieces

6 cups water or homemade bone broth

2 cups bok choy, chopped

1 tbsp sea salt

1 tbsp fresh herbs (optional – parsley, cilantro) for garnish

Ginger-Scallion Poached Chicken

1. In a large pot, place the whole chicken and cover with 6 cups of water or bone broth. Add the sliced ginger and chopped scallions. Bring to a boil over medium-high heat.

2. Once the broth is boiling, reduce the heat to low and let the chicken simmer for 1-1.5 hours, or until the chicken is fully cooked and tender. Skim off any impurities or foam that rises to the surface.

3. In the last 10 minutes of cooking, add the chopped bok choy to the pot and let it wilt in the broth.

4. Remove the chicken from the pot and carve it. Serve the chicken pieces with the bok choy and ladle the broth over the top. Garnish with fresh herbs if desired.

Sage and Apple Turkey Meatballs

Prep Time: 15 minutes

Cook Time: 30-35 minutes (for spaghetti squash) + 10 minutes (for meatballs)

Servings: 3-4

Ingredients:

1 lb ground turkey

1 medium apple, grated (skin on)

2 tbsp fresh sage, finely chopped

2 cloves garlic, minced

½ small onion, finely chopped

1 egg (optional, for binding)

½ tsp sea salt

¼ tsp black pepper (omit for AIP)

2 tbsp olive oil

1 small spaghetti squash, roasted

1. In a bowl, combine ground turkey, grated apple, sage, garlic, onion, egg (if using), sea salt, and black pepper. Mix well until fully combined.

2. Shape the mixture into 1-inch meatballs.

3. Heat olive oil in a skillet over medium heat. Add the meatballs and cook, turning occasionally, for 8-10 minutes, until golden brown and cooked through (internal temperature should reach 165°F or 74°C).

4. While the meatballs are cooking, roast the spaghetti squash. Cut in half lengthwise, scoop out seeds, drizzle with olive oil, and season with a pinch of salt. Roast at 400°F (200°C) for 30-35 minutes or until tender. Use a fork to shred the squash into strands.

5. Serve the sage and apple turkey meatballs over the roasted spaghetti squash.

Prep Time: 15 minutes

Cook Time: 1 hour 15 minutes

Servings: 4

Ingredients:

1 lb cubed grass-fed beef

4 cups homemade bone broth (beef or chicken)

2 medium carrots, diced

2 celery stalks, diced

1 onion, chopped

2 sprigs fresh thyme

2 bay leaves

2 medium sweet potatoes, peeled and diced

½ tsp sea salt

¼ tsp black pepper (omit for AIP)

Grass-Fed Beef Bone Broth Stew

1. Heat a large pot over medium-high heat. Add a little olive oil, then add the cubed beef. Brown the meat on all sides (about 5-7 minutes).

2. Add the diced onions, carrots, and celery to the pot. Sauté for about 3-4 minutes until the vegetables start to soften.

3. Pour in the bone broth, add thyme, bay leaves, salt, and pepper, and stir to combine.

4. Bring the stew to a boil, then reduce the heat to low. Let it simmer for 45-60 minutes, or until the beef is tender and the vegetables are cooked through.

5. Stir in the diced sweet potatoes and cook for an additional 20-25 minutes, or until the sweet potatoes are fork-tender.

6. Remove the bay leaves and thyme sprigs. Ladle the stew into bowls and serve warm.

Prep Time: 10-15 minutes

Cook Time: 20-30 minutes

Servings: 2

Ingredients:

4 grass-fed lamb chops

2 tbsp fresh rosemary, chopped

3 cloves garlic, minced

2 tbsp olive oil (for the lamb)

1 lb Brussels sprouts, trimmed and halved

1 tbsp olive oil

½ tsp sea salt

¼ tsp black pepper (omit for AIP)

1 lemon

Garlic-Rosemary Lamb Chops

1. Preheat the oven to 400°F (200°C). Toss the halved Brussels sprouts with 1 tbsp olive oil, salt, and pepper. Spread them evenly on a baking sheet and roast for 20-25 minutes, or until they are golden and crispy on the edges, shaking the pan halfway through.

2. In a small bowl, combine the minced garlic, fresh rosemary, 2 tbsp olive oil, and a pinch of sea salt. Rub the mixture all over the lamb chops. Let them marinate for at least 10 minutes (or up to 30 minutes in the fridge).

3. Heat a grill pan or skillet over medium-high heat. Cook the lamb chops for about 4-5 minutes per side for medium-rare, or longer for desired doneness. Remove from heat and let rest for a few minutes before serving.

4. Plate the lamb chops and serve with the roasted Brussels sprouts. Garnish with a squeeze of fresh lemon juice, if desired.

Sue Slaughter

Prep Time: 10 minutes

Cook Time: 15 minutes

Servings: 2

Ingredients:

8 oz thinly sliced grass-fed beef (sirloin or flank steak)

1-inch piece fresh ginger, grated

2 cloves garlic, minced

2 tbsp lime juice (freshly squeezed)

2 tbsp coconut aminos

1 cup broccoli florets

1 cup carrots, thinly sliced

1 cup bok choy, chopped

2 tbsp olive oil

2 cups cauliflower rice

Ginger-Lime Beef Stir-Fry

1. In a skillet, heat 1 tbsp olive oil over medium heat. Add cauliflower rice and sauté for 5-7 minutes, until soft and slightly golden. Set aside.

2. In a large skillet or wok, heat 1 tbsp olive oil over medium-high heat. Add the sliced beef and stir-fry for 3-4 minutes until browned. Remove from the skillet and set aside.

3. In the same skillet, add garlic and ginger. Sauté for 1-2 minutes until fragrant.

4. Add the broccoli, carrots, and bok choy to the skillet and stir-fry for 3-4 minutes until tender-crisp.

5. Return the beef to the skillet. Add lime juice and coconut aminos, stirring to combine. Cook for an additional 2-3 minutes until the sauce thickens slightly.

6. Plate the stir-fry over a bed of cauliflower rice and garnish with extra lime slices or fresh herbs if desired.

Moroccan Lamb Stew

Prep Time: 10 minutes

Cook Time: 55 minutes

Servings: 4

Ingredients:

1 lb cubed lamb shoulder (preferably grass-fed)

2 tbsp olive oil

1 tsp ground turmeric

1 tsp ground cinnamon

1 tsp ground ginger

2 large sweet potatoes, peeled and cubed

3 carrots, peeled and sliced

4 cups homemade bone broth (chicken or beef)

1 tbsp fresh parsley, chopped (for garnish)

1 small head of cauliflower, grated or processed into couscous-sized pieces

1 tbsp olive oil

½ tsp sea salt

¼ tsp black pepper (omit for AIP)

1. In a large pot or Dutch oven, heat olive oil over medium heat. Add cubed lamb and brown on all sides, about 5-7 minutes.

2. Stir in turmeric, cinnamon, and ginger, and cook for another minute to release their aromas.

3. Add sweet potatoes, carrots, and bone broth to the pot. Bring the mixture to a boil, then reduce heat to low and simmer for 40-45 minutes, or until the lamb is tender and the vegetables are cooked through.

4. While the stew is simmering, heat 1 tbsp olive oil in a skillet over medium heat. Add the cauliflower couscous and sauté for 5-7 minutes, stirring occasionally, until tender and slightly golden. Season with salt and pepper to taste.

5. Ladle the lamb stew into bowls, serve with cauliflower couscous on the side, and garnish with fresh parsley.

Herb-Crusted Rack of Lamb

Prep Time: 10 minutes

Cook Time: 25-30 minutes

Servings: 4

Ingredients:

1 rack of grass-fed lamb (about 8 ribs)

2 tbsp fresh thyme, chopped

2 tbsp fresh rosemary, chopped

3 cloves garlic, minced

2 tbsp olive oil

1 tbsp olive oil

1 bulb fennel, sliced

3 medium carrots, peeled and sliced

1 tsp sea salt (divided)

½ tsp black pepper (omit for AIP)

1 lemon, sliced

1. Preheat your oven to 400°F (200°C). In a small bowl, mix chopped thyme, rosemary, garlic, 2 tbsp olive oil, salt, and pepper. Rub this herb mixture evenly over the rack of lamb.

2. Heat a skillet over medium-high heat. Sear the lamb rack for 2-3 minutes on each side until golden brown.

3. Transfer the lamb to a baking sheet and roast in the preheated oven for 15-20 minutes for medium-rare (adjust time for desired doneness). Let it rest for 5-10 minutes before slicing.

4. While the lamb is roasting, toss sliced fennel and carrots with 1 tbsp olive oil, sea salt, and black pepper. Spread them on a baking sheet and roast in the oven for 20-25 minutes until tender and caramelized.

5. Slice the rack of lamb between the bones and serve with the roasted fennel and carrots. Garnish with lemon slices for extra freshness.

Slow-Cooked Beef Short Ribs with Mashed Cauliflower

Prep Time: 10 minutes

Cook Time: 7-8 hours (slow cooker) or 4-5 hours (high setting)

Servings: 4-6

Ingredients:

4-6 grass-fed beef short ribs

2 cups bone broth (beef or chicken)

1 large onion, chopped

2 carrots, chopped

2 celery stalks, chopped

3 cloves garlic, minced

2-3 fresh thyme sprigs

2 bay leaves

1 tbsp olive oil

1 head cauliflower, chopped into florets

1 tbsp olive oil or ghee

½ tsp sea salt

¼ tsp black pepper (omit for AIP)

1. Heat olive oil in a large skillet over medium-high heat. Season the short ribs with sea salt and black pepper. Sear the ribs on all sides for 3-4 minutes, until browned.

2. Transfer the seared short ribs to a slow cooker. Add onion, carrots, celery, garlic, thyme, bay leaves, and bone broth.

3. Cover and cook on low for 7-8 hours or on high for 4-5 hours, until the short ribs are tender and falling off the bone.

4. While the ribs cook, steam the cauliflower florets until tender (about 10-12 minutes).

5. In a bowl, mash the cauliflower with olive oil or ghee, sea salt, and black pepper (omit black pepper for AIP).

6. Remove the short ribs from the slow cooker and serve with a generous helping of mashed cauliflower.

Sue Slaughter

Bison Burger Bowls

Prep Time: 10 minutes

Cook Time: 12 minutes

Servings: 4

Ingredients:

1 lb ground bison (for 4 patties)

2 cups mixed greens like spinach, arugula, or kale

1 avocado, sliced

1 cup mushrooms, sliced

½ onion, thinly sliced

2 tbsp olive oil (divided)

1 tbsp lemon juice

Sea salt and black pepper (to taste, omit black pepper for AIP)

1. Form the ground bison into 4 equal patties, seasoning with a pinch of sea salt and black pepper (omit black pepper for AIP).

2. Heat 1 tablespoon of olive oil in a pan over medium heat. Cook the bison patties for 4-5 minutes per side, or until browned and cooked through. Set aside.

3. In the same pan, add another tablespoon of olive oil. Sauté the mushrooms and onions for 4-5 minutes until softened and slightly caramelized.

4. In serving bowls, layer the mixed greens, avocado slices, sautéed mushrooms and onions, and bison patties.

5. Drizzle with olive oil and lemon juice, and season with salt and pepper.

Honey-Garlic Pork Tenderloin

Prep Time: 10 minutes

Cook Time: 30-35 minutes

Servings: 4

Ingredients:

1 pasture-raised pork tenderloin (about 1 lb)

2 tbsp raw honey

4 cloves garlic, minced

2 tbsp coconut aminos

2 medium sweet potatoes, cubed

2 apples, cored and sliced

1 tbsp olive oil

½ tsp sea salt

¼ tsp black pepper (omit for AIP)

1 tsp fresh rosemary or thyme

1. Preheat the oven to 400°F (200°C). In a small bowl, combine raw honey, minced garlic, and coconut aminos. Stir well.

2. Heat 1 tbsp olive oil in an oven-safe skillet over medium-high heat. Sear the pork tenderloin on all sides until browned, about 3-4 minutes.

3. Brush the honey-garlic sauce over the pork tenderloin, making sure to coat it evenly.

4. Transfer the skillet to the preheated oven and roast the pork for 20-25 minutes, or until the internal temperature reaches 145°F (63°C).

5. While the pork is roasting, toss the cubed sweet potatoes and apple slices with olive oil, sea salt, and black pepper (optional). Spread them in a single layer on a baking sheet and roast in the oven for 25-30 minutes, or until tender and slightly caramelized, stirring halfway through.

6. Once the pork is done, remove it from the oven and let it rest for 5 minutes before slicing. Serve with the roasted sweet potatoes and apples.

Prep Time: 15 minutes

Cook Time: 2.5 hours

Servings: 2

Ingredients:

2 grass-fed lamb shanks

4 cloves garlic, minced

2 tbsp fresh rosemary, chopped

2 cups bone broth (chicken or beef)

2 tbsp olive oil

1 tsp sea salt

½ tsp black pepper (omit for AIP)

4 large parsnips, peeled and chopped

1 tbsp olive oil

¼ tsp sea salt

½ cup coconut milk

Rosemary-Garlic Lamb Shanks with Mashed Parsnips

1. Preheat the oven to 325°F (165°C). Season the lamb shanks with sea salt and black pepper.

2. Heat olive oil in a large ovenproof pot over medium-high heat. Sear the lamb shanks on all sides until browned, about 4-5 minutes.

3. Add minced garlic and chopped rosemary to the pot and cook for 1 minute until fragrant.

4. Pour in the bone broth and bring to a simmer. Cover the pot with a lid and transfer to the preheated oven. Braise for 2-2.5 hours, or until the lamb is fork-tender.

5. While the lamb cooks, bring a pot of water to a boil and add the parsnips. Cook for 12-15 minutes, or until tender. Drain, then mash with olive oil, sea salt, and coconut milk (if using) until smooth and creamy.

6. Plate the lamb shanks with mashed parsnips and spoon some of the braising liquid over the top. Garnish with additional fresh rosemary if desired.

4-Week Anti-Inflammatory Diet Plan

Week 1

Day 1
- Breakfast: Berry Turmeric Smoothie (p.27)
- Lunch: Wild Salmon and Avocado Salad (p.48)
- Dinner: Turmeric Ginger Chicken Thighs with Cauliflower Rice (p.110)

Day 2
- Breakfast: Coconut Yogurt Parfait (p.38)
- Lunch: Stuffed Portobello Mushrooms (p.75)
- Dinner: Moroccan Lamb Stew (p.63)

Day 3
- Breakfast: Carrot Cake Smoothie (p.32)
- Lunch: Mediterranean Stuffed Sweet Potatoes (p.78)
- Dinner: Herb-Roasted Wild Salmon with Lemon (p.90)

Day 4
- Breakfast: Breakfast Bowl (p.39)
- Lunch: Zucchini Noodle Stir-Fry (p.73)
- Dinner: Ginger-Poached Cod with Bok Choy (p.91)

Day 5
- Breakfast: Avocado Mint Smoothie (p.31)
- Lunch: Sweet Potato Avocado Bites (p.53)
- Dinner: Bison Burger Bowls (p.125)

Day 6
- Breakfast: Sautéed Greens with Poached Eggs (p.41)
- Lunch: Sardine and Cucumber Salad (p.104)
- Dinner: Coconut Curry Chicken with Cauliflower Rice (p.113)

Day 7
- Breakfast: Fig and Blackberry Smoothie (p.33)
- Lunch: Roasted Vegetable Tian with Pine Nuts (p.74)
- Dinner: Grass-Fed Beef Bone Broth Stew (p.119)

Sue Slaughter

Week 2

Day 1
- Breakfast: Green Smoothie (p.28)
- Lunch: Tropical Kale and Mango Salad (p.49)
- Dinner: Lemon Herb Turkey Burgers (p.111)

Day 2
- Breakfast: Sweet Potato Boats (p.44)
- Lunch: Zucchini Pasta with Avocado Cream Sauce (p.86)
- Dinner: Herbed Scallops with Roasted Root Vegetables (p.96)

Day 3
- Breakfast: Turmeric Chia Pudding (p.35)
- Lunch: Spaghetti Squash Pad Thai (p.83)
- Dinner: Slow-Cooked Beef Short Ribs with Mashed Cauliflower (p.124)

Day 4
- Breakfast: Sweet Potato Pie Smoothie (p.34)
- Lunch: Cucumber Sushi Rolls (p.55)
- Dinner: Apple Cider Vinegar Chicken with Roasted Root Vegetables (p.112)

Day 5
- Breakfast: Herbal Congee (p.46)
- Lunch: Warm Brussels Sprout and Apple Salad (p.88)
- Dinner: Miso-Glazed Black Cod (p.93)

Day 6
- Breakfast: Breakfast Porridge (p.40)
- Lunch: Stuffed Acorn Squash with Wild Rice & Mushrooms (p.72)
- Dinner: Garlic-Rosemary Lamb Chops (p.120)

Day 7
- Breakfast: Tropical Turmeric Smoothie (p.30)
- Lunch: Warm Quinoa and Roasted Vegetable Bowl (p.82)
- Dinner: Coconut-Poached Halibut (p.95)

Week 3

Day 1
- Breakfast: Cherry Ginger Smoothie (p.29)

- Lunch: Zucchini Herb Fritters with Coconut Yogurt (p.56)
- Dinner: Rosemary Balsamic Chicken with Roasted Brussels Sprouts (p.116)

Day 2
- Breakfast: Berry and Coconut Bowl (p.45)
- Lunch: Cauliflower Steaks with Herb Sauce (p.80)
- Dinner: Tuna Steak with Ginger-Scallion Sauce (p.98)

Day 3
- Breakfast: Butternut Squash Bowl (p.42)
- Lunch: Sweet Potato Hash (p.37)
- Dinner: Honey-Garlic Pork Tenderloin (p.126)

Day 4
- Breakfast: Carrot Cake Smoothie (p.32)
- Lunch: Wild Mushroom Risotto with Cauliflower Rice (p.71)
- Dinner: Sage and Apple Turkey Meatballs (p.118)

Day 5
- Breakfast: Avocado Mint Smoothie (p.31)
- Lunch: Sardine and Cucumber Toast (p.43)
- Dinner: Seafood and Sweet Potato Stew (p.99)

Day 6
- Breakfast: Fig and Blackberry Smoothie (p.33)
- Lunch: Summer Roll Bowls (p.81)
- Dinner: Baked Sole with Herb Crust and Sautéed Zucchini Noodles (p.92)

Day 7
- Breakfast: Sweet Potato Pie Smoothie (p.34)
- Lunch: Roasted Root Vegetable Salad (p.50)
- Dinner: Ginger-Lime Beef Stir-Fry (p.121)

Week 4

Day 1
- Breakfast: Green Smoothie (p.28)
- Lunch: Wild Blueberry Spinach Salad (p.51)
- Dinner: Baked Mackerel with Herbs (p.97)

Day 2
- Breakfast: Turmeric Chia Pudding (p.35)
- Lunch: Spaghetti Squash with Basil-Avocado Pesto (p.76)
- Dinner: Ginger-Scallion Poached Chicken (p.117)

Day 3
- Breakfast: Berry Turmeric Smoothie (p.27)
- Lunch: Maple-Glazed Root Vegetables with Cauliflower Mash (p.85)
- Dinner: Herb-Crusted Rack of Lamb (p.123)

Day 4
- Breakfast: Coconut Yogurt Parfait (p.38)
- Lunch: Scallop and Cucumber Noodle Salad (p.107)
- Dinner: Citrus Herb Cornish Game Hens (p.115)

Day 5
- Breakfast: Carrot Cake Smoothie (p.32)
- Lunch: Baked Stuffed Avocados with Crab (p.108)
- Dinner: Cioppino-Inspired Seafood Soup (p.101)

Day 6
- Breakfast: Butternut Squash Bowl (p.42)
- Lunch: Shrimp and Avocado Lettuce Cups (p.102)
- Dinner: Rosemary-Garlic Lamb Shanks with Mashed Parsnips (p.127)

Day 7
- Breakfast: Sweet Potato Boats (p.44)
- Lunch: Seafood and Avocado Ceviche (p.105)
- Dinner: Wild Salmon and Fennel Soup (p.100)

Recipe Index

Sue Slaughter

- Seafood and Sweet Potato Stew – 99
- Shrimp and Avocado Lettuce Cups – 102
- Slow-Cooked Beef Short Ribs with Mashed Cauliflower – 124
- Smoked Salmon Bowl – 103
- Spaghetti Squash Pad Thai – 83
- Spaghetti Squash with Basil-Avocado Pesto – 76
- Stuffed Acorn Squash with Wild Rice & Mushrooms – 72
- Stuffed Collard Green Wraps – 84
- Stuffed Mushroom Caps with Spinach – 57
- Stuffed Portobello Mushrooms – 75
- Summer Roll Bowls – 81
- Sweet Potato Avocado Bites – 53
- Sweet Potato Boats – 44
- Sweet Potato Breakfast Hash – 37
- Sweet Potato Pie Smoothie – 34

T
- Tropical Kale and Mango Salad – 49
- Tropical Turmeric Smoothie – 30
- Tuna Steak with Ginger-Scallion Sauce – 98
- Turmeric Cauliflower Bites – 54
- Turmeric Chia Pudding – 35
- Turmeric Ginger Chicken Thighs with Cauliflower Rice – 110
- Turmeric Sauce – 67

W
- Warm Brussels Sprout and Apple Salad – 88
- Warm Quinoa and Roasted Vegetable Bowl – 82
- Wild Blueberry Spinach Salad – 51
- Wild Mushroom and Asparagus Risotto – 87
- Wild Mushroom Risotto with Cauliflower Rice – 71
- Wild Salmon and Avocado Salad – 48
- Wild Salmon and Fennel Soup – 100
- Wild Salmon Chowder – 61

Z
- Zucchini Herb Fritters with Coconut Yogurt – 56
- Zucchini Noodle Stir-Fry – 73
- Zucchini Pasta with Avocado Cream Sauce – 86

Sue Slaughter

Made in the USA
Columbia, SC
27 April 2025

57218576R00076